ABC of
Emergency Radiology

Second Edition

ABC series

The revised and updated ABC series – written by specialists for non-specialists

- With over 40 titles, this extensive series provides a quick and dependable reference on a broad range of topics in all the major specialities

- An easy-to-use resource, covering the symptoms, investigations, treatment and management of conditions presenting in your day-to-day practice

- Full colour photographs and illustrations aid diagnosis and patient understanding of a condition

- Each book in the new series now offers links to further information and articles, and a new dedicated website provides even more support

- A highly illustrated, informative and practical source of knowledge for GPs, GP registrars, junior doctors, doctors in training and those in primary care

For further information on the entire ABC series, please visit:

www.abcbookseries.com

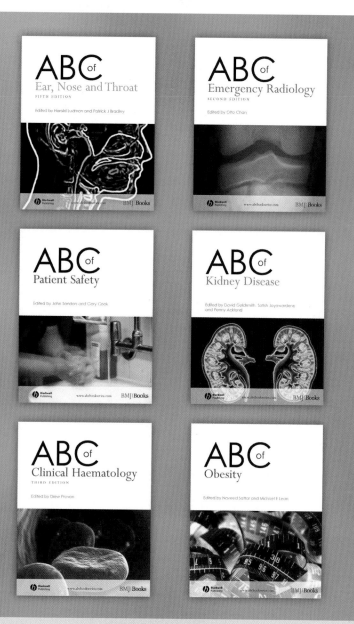

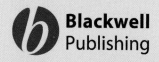

Blackwell Publishing

BMJ|Books

ABC of Emergency Radiology

Second Edition

EDITED BY

Otto Chan

Consultant Radiologist, The London Independent Hospital, London, UK

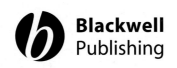

Blackwell
Publishing

BMJ | Books

© Blackwell Publishing Ltd 2007

BMJ Books is an imprint of the BMJ Publishing Group, used under licence

Blackwell Publishing Inc., 350 Main Street, Malden, Massachusetts 02148-5020, USA
Blackwell Publishing Ltd, 9600 Garsington Road, Oxford OX4 2DQ, UK
Blackwell Publishing Asia Pty Ltd, 550 Swanston Street, Carlton, Victoria 3053, Australia

The right of the Author to be identified as the Author of the Work has been asserted in
accordance with the Copyright, Designs and Patents Act 1988.

All rights reserved. No part of this publication may be reproduced, stored in a
retrieval system, or transmitted, in any form or by any means, electronic, mechanical,
photocopying, recording and/or otherwise, except as permitted by the UK Copyright,
Designs and Patents Act 1988, without the prior written permission of the publisher.

First edition 1995
Second edition 2007

1 2007

Library of Congress Cataloging-in-Publication Data
ABC of emergency radiology. -- 2nd ed. / edited by Otto Chan.
    p. ; cm.
    Includes bibliographical references and index.
    ISBN-13: 978-0-7279-1528-3
    ISBN-10: 0-7279-1528-2
    1. Radiography, Medical. 2. Emergency medicine--Diagnosis. I. Chan, Otto.
    [DNLM: 1. Radiography. 2. Emergencies. WN 200 A134 2007]

    RC78.A562 2007
    616.07'572--dc22

                                                       2006103167

ISBN: 978-0-7279-1528-3

A catalogue record for this book is available from the British Library

The cover shows avulsion of the anterior cruciate ligament and is used with permission of
Otto Chan

Set in 9.25/12 pt Minion by Sparks, Oxford – www.sparks.co.uk
Printed and bound at GraphyCems, Navarra, Spain

Commissioning Editor: Mary Banks
Editorial Assistant: Victoria Pittman
Development Editor: Sally Carter / Vicki Donald
Production Controller: Rachel Edwards

For further information on Blackwell Publishing, visit our website:
www.blackwellpublishing.com

The publisher's policy is to use permanent paper from mills that operate a sustainable
forestry policy, and which has been manufactured from pulp processed using acid-free and
elementary chlorine-free practices. Furthermore, the publisher ensures that the text paper
and cover board used have met acceptable environmental accreditation standards.

Blackwell Publishing makes no representation, express or implied, that the drug dosages
in this book are correct. Readers must therefore always check that any product mentioned
in this publication is used in accordance with the prescribing information prepared by the
manufacturers. The author and the publishers do not accept responsibility or legal liability
for any errors in the text or for the misuse or misapplication of material in this book.

DATE 21.06.07
ACC. No. 009993
CLASS No. 616.0757 CHA

Contents

Contributors

Muaaze Ahmad
Consultant Musculoskeletal Radiologist, Barts and The Royal London NHS Trust, London

Laurence H Berman
Ultrasound Consultant, Addenbrooke's Hospital, Cambridge

Roger N Bodley
Consultant Radiologist, Stoke Mandeville Hospital, Buckinghamshire

Otto Chan
Consultant Radiologist, The London Independent Hospital, London

Gerald de Lacey
Consultant Radiologist, Radiology Red Dot Courses, London

Marina J Easty
Consultant in Paediatric Radiology, Great Ormond Street Hospital, London

David A Elias
Consultant Radiologist, King's College Hospital, London

Rashika Fernando
Specialist Registrar in Diagnostic Radiology, King's College Hospital, London

Tim Fotheringham
Consultant Interventional Radiologist, The Royal London Hospital, London

Simon Holmes
Consultant Maxillofacial Surgeon, The Royal London Hospital, London

Tudor H Hughes
Associate Professor of Radiology, University of California San Diego, USA

Rosy Jalan
Consultant Paediatric Radiologist, Royal London Hospital, London

Andreas Koureas
Lecturer, University of Athens, Athens, Greece

Paula McAlinden
Consultant Radiologist, Royal Bournemouth Hospital, Bournemouth

Amrish Mehta
Consultant Neuroradiologist, Charing Cross Hospital, London

Ali Naraghi
Assistant Professor of Radiology, Mount Sinai Hospital and University Health Network, University of Toronto, Toronto, Canada

Caroline C Parlier-Cuau
Hôpital Lariboisière, Paris, France

Niall Power
Consultant Radiologist, Royal London Hospital, London

Peter Renton (deceased)
Formerly Consultant Radiologist, University College Hospital London

Lee F Rogers
Professor, University of Arizona Health Sciences Center, Tucson, Arizona, USA

May-ai Seah
Specialist Registrar in Diagnostic Radiology, King's College Hospital, London

Kathirkamanathan Shanmuganathan
Professor, Department of Diagnostic Radiology, University of Maryland School of Medicine, Baltimore, USA

Clint W Sliker
Assistant Professor, University of Maryland Medical School, Baltimore, USA

James Teh
Consultant Radiologist, Nuffield Orthopaedic Centre, Oxford

Robin Touquet
Consultant in Emergency Medicine, St Mary's Hospital, London

Michael Walsh
Consultant Trauma and Vascular Surgeon, The Royal London Hospital, London

Alastair Wilson
Consultant in Accident and Emergency, The Royal London Hospital, London

James A S Young
Specialist Registrar in Radiology, Barts and The Royal London NHS Trust, London

Jeremy W R Young
DISC Imaging, Mount Pleasant SC United States

Preface

There have been dramatic technological advances in diagnostic imaging over the past two decades, but the rapid acquisition and interpretation of plain radiographic images remains the mainstay of initial successful management of sick or traumatised patients in accident and emergency departments.

Virtually any medical condition can present to accident and emergency departments, and so the volume of medical knowledge needed to manage these patients satisfactorily is enormous. It is unfortunate that most of these patients are initially seen and treated by relatively inexperienced staff – usually medical students, house officers, senior house officers, specialist registrars, or nurses – who often have had little or no training in the interpretation of plain radiographs.

Rapid and accurate interpretation of these radiographs is often the key to quick and correct management of patients in the accident and emergency department. Although safety nets exist, specialist radiological advice is often not available at the time of presentation – when it is most needed. Staff in the accident and emergency department who manage these patients need to be able to interpret these radiographs for quick, accurate, and effective initial treatment, to avoid errors in interpretation, inappropriate treatment, and medicolegal consequences.

The authors of the *ABC of Emergency Radiology* have produced a simple and logical step by step approach on how to interpret radiographs. The book is divided into anatomical regions and followed by chapters in paediatrics and major trauma. The chapters start with normal basic radiological anatomy, followed by the standard radiographs, then a simple ABCs systematic approach on basic interpretation of the radiographs, a review of abnormalities, and a summary.

This book provides a simple, concise, and systematic approach to the interpretation of plain radiographs. It should be very helpful to medical students, foundation doctors, specialist registrars, and consultants in all specialties, and also other health professionals working in accident and emergency, in particular radiographers and nurses.

Otto Chan

To my family.

General Aspects of Trauma

Lee F Rogers

Trauma was long regarded as a subject unworthy of study and research in medicine. The serious collective morbidity and mortality caused by trauma has now been acknowledged, and the enormous collective costs of the initial treatment and subsequent care have been computed and tabulated. The numbers are large. As a result, trauma is now a matter of conscious concern to the medical profession and government at all levels. Trauma is finally receiving the attention it deserves.

In 1966, publication of the landmark white paper, *Accidental death and disability, the neglected disease of modern society*, by the National Academy of Sciences showed the full impact of trauma. It resulted in dramatic changes. Guidelines were published to establish regionalised trauma care, and they have been adopted widely in the United States. Anderson and colleagues carried out a similar study in the United Kingdom, and this has led to a sea change in the management of trauma in the United Kingdom. The introduction of advanced trauma life support training has been of great importance. Where adopted and implemented, specialised trauma centres have substantially improved the care of the injured. The need for research into trauma is vital because of its effect on the quality of life of people who have sustained trauma injuries and because of the high cost of treatment (more than $20 billion a year in the United States alone).

Epidemiology of trauma

Trauma can occur to anyone at any time. Skeletal injuries occur during the course of all human activities. The expectation and risk of injury varies with the nature of the endeavour. Nobody is immune, irrespective of age, sex, activity, or state of health. Trauma is unexpected and sudden. At best, an injury may cause a minor degree of inconvenience; at worst, it can cause death. Before the event, those affected may have been in excellent health. In the next moment, life may hang precariously in the balance. Of course, criminal activities, assaults, and beatings result in skeletal injury, but no human activity is free of the risk of injury. Even mundane activities in the home, at work, or at play carry a finite risk.

Repetitive activities in industrial settings lend themselves to analysis, and preventive measures can be taken to reduce the incidence of injury. In other situations, effective preventive measures have been identified, but they have been only partially accepted by the public. Laws have long been in place that set speed limits, prohibit driving

Trauma

- Common
- Major cause of morbidity and mortality
- Expensive to treat
- Treatment poorly funded

Prevention and minimisation of accidents are now recognised as important contributions to people's lives, as well as a means of reducing healthcare expenditure

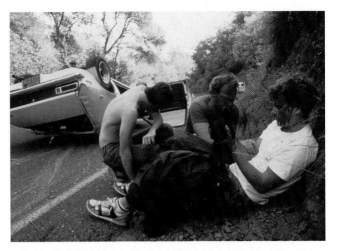

Injuries and death associated with motor vehicle crashes at high speed have reached plague-like proportions. With permission from Peter Menzel/Science Photo Library.

Motorcyclists are 13 times more likely to die in a road traffic crash than drivers of cars, even though it has been shown repeatedly that the use of helmets reduces head injury, death, and disability in motorcyclists

while under the influence of alcohol, and mandate the use seat belts, yet many people ignore these laws and are a menace to themselves and others.

Frequency and distribution of fractures

The location, nature, and number of fractures depend on the age of the individual, the nature and severity of the trauma, and the status of the skeletal system.

The activity in which a person is engaged when injured can be predicated by their age. The young will probably be injured in the course of play or sports activities. Mature adults (aged 20-50 years) are more likely to sustain an injury while travelling in a motor vehicle or at work. Falls are more often a source of injury in elderly people than other causes, including motor vehicle crashes. Many elderly people are sedentary, often affected by osteoporosis, and more likely to be injured in a fall during the course of normal activities – for example, walking, descending stairs, stepping from a curb, or moving about in a bathroom.

Fatalities in trauma

In the developed world, injuries are the leading cause of death for more than half of the human life span (1-43 years). Trauma is the fourth most common cause of death after heart disease, cancer, and stroke. About 150 000 US citizens of all ages die from trauma each year, and about a third of these deaths are from motor vehicle crashes. Motor vehicle crashes are the leading cause of death between the ages of 5 and 34 years.

The World Health Organization (WHO) has estimated that in the year 2000, 1.26 million people worldwide died from road traffic crashes. Injuries outnumber all other causes of death in children and young adults. Almost half of all deaths in US children are the result of trauma. Crashes involving motor cars and children who are pedestrians are the leading source of multiple injuries in children. Such incidents are followed distantly by motor vehicle crashes with children as passengers, crashes involving children on bicycles and motor vehicle crashes involving motor cycles, and falls from great heights. Children tend to survive multiple injuries more often than adults.

The overall death rate of those who sustain multiple injuries is about 10-25%. People >70 years are affected more severely by accidents than those from other age groups. Trauma is the fifth leading cause of death in patients >65 years. Although people in this age group are less likely to be injured than those in younger age groups, older individuals are more likely to die from their injuries. In older people, mortality from accidents is five times higher than that in younger people.

Initial evaluation of injured people

The first two steps in the care of an injured person should be a carefully performed medical history and physical examination. An evaluation of the airway and checks for the presence of shock, haemorrhage, and open wounds are essential. In each of these areas, corrective measures must be taken immediately if necessary. Fractures

> The skeleton is weak when immature, at maximum strength when mature, and weakened by age. Regardless of age, the strength of the skeleton is diminished by disease (metastases or rheumatoid arthritis), and by hormonal imbalances of renal disease, rickets, scurvy, Cushing's disease, diabetes, and exogenous steroids

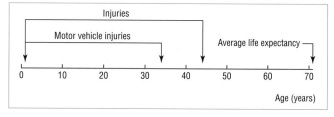

The portion of the average life span during which injuries are the main cause of death in the United States. Adapted from Baker SP. Injuries: The neglected epidemic. Stone Lecture 1985. American Trauma Society Meeting. *J Trauma* 1987;27:343.

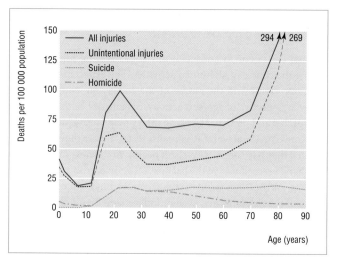

Death rates in the United States for injuries by age, 1930-1980. Adapted from Baker SP. Injuries: The neglected epidemic. Stone Lecture 1985. American Trauma Society Meeting. *J Trauma* 1987;27:343

should be noted and splints applied. These actions will assist in the handling of the patient and reduce morbidity in seriously injured patients.

The physical examination of comatose patients or patients with multiple injuries (often seen in patients from vehicle accidents) is difficult because the patient is unable to cooperate or respond to queries. Injuries can be easily overlooked, which heightens the importance of imaging.

Radiographic examination should never be considered a substitute for taking a patient's history and doing a physical examination. Serious injuries can often exist even if they are not found on a radiograph.

Imaging to assess injured people

Successful treatment of skeletal injury starts with accurate diagnosis. A good history and physical examination, and to ensure the patient is haemodynamically stable is necessary for this. Then the patient needs a well performed and accurately interpreted radiographic examination. The standard views for radiographs have been adopted because they show most abnormalities. Failing to obtain all of the standard views heightens the chance for oversights and diagnostic errors.

A radiographic examination to exclude a skeletal injury of any anatomical part should never be obtained in a single plane only. Radiographs obtained in two planes at right angles are the minimum, and radiographic examinations of joints need additional oblique views to exclude fractures and dislocations. Patients who have severe trauma require computed tomography to identify or exclude injuries of the central nervous system, vascular area, chest, and intra-abdominal visceral injuries, as well as injuries of the face skeleton, spine, and pelvis.

The physician or radiologist's interpretation of a radiographic examination (or any type of imaging examination) is facilitated greatly by an appropriate history on the request form. Unfortunately, the history being included for the radiologist can be perfunctory, incomplete, or even misleading. The lack of a good history compromises the radiologist's evaluation. The history should state precisely where the patient hurts and the initial clinical impression – for example, "Pain in snuff box, rule out fracture of the scaphoid." Knowledge of where the patient hurts directs attention to the area of principal clinical concern and, at the same time, steers the radiologist away from questionable findings in other parts of the film that have no clinical importance.

Injuries are repetitive. That is to say, in each anatomical part injuries occur at some sites more often than at others. People who interpret radiographs of patients with trauma should be aware of the sites of the most common injuries in each anatomical part. They should exclude injuries at those specific sites. For example, with pain in the wrist – epiphyseal fractures of the distal radius should be excluded in adolescents, scaphoid and triquetral fractures are most common in young adults, and Colles' fractures should be looked for in elderly people.

> To the patient, the prime concern of personnel in an emergency department can seem to be paperwork, proof of insurance, and many other matters unrelated to the patient's injury. Every doctor should be concerned about the apparent, or actual, need for prolonged administrative questioning about the evaluation and care of patients

> The radiographic examination should never be considered a substitute for a patient's history and physical examination

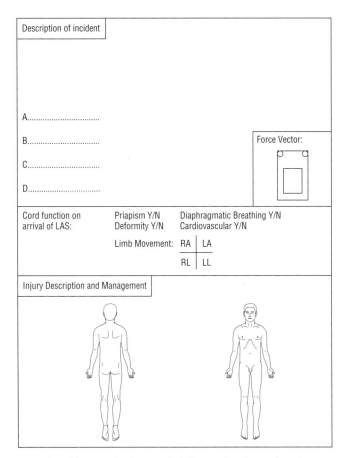

In a patient's history, a simple anatomical diagram that shows where the patient hurts, clearly marked in pen or pencil by the doctor, is extremely helpful. This figure is adapted from a patient assessment form for use by staff working in fast response vehicles.

Soft tissue signs that point to underlying injury of the bone and joint should be specifically identified or excluded. These include the fat pad sign at the elbow joint, which indicates haemoarthrosis, and the fat-fluid sign at the knee, which alerts the doctor to an intra-articular fracture of the knee joint.

KEY POINTS

- Traumatic injury is common at all ages and is the leading cause of death in children and young adults
- Imaging plays a key role in the evaluation and treatment of injured people
- Prompt and accurate identification of injuries assures appropriate treatment, thus reducing the morbidity and mortality of those injured. This is a worthy goal for all involved in their care

CHAPTER 1

General Principles: How to Interpret Radiographs

Otto Chan, Robin Touquet

Emergency medicine often brings together critically ill patients with inexperienced junior doctors – a dangerous combination with potentially serious consequences. The huge volume of information necessary to manage these patients adequately is overwhelming, as virtually any condition can present itself. The difficulties are compounded because radiographs are requested for many patients. These radiographs may be interpreted by relatively inexperienced, and often tired, personnel who have little training in how to evaluate them.

Radiographic projections

Site	View	Comment
Finger	Anteroposterior and lateral	
Hand	Anteroposterior and oblique	
Wrist	Anteroposterior and lateral	Four views for suspected scaphoid fractures
Elbow	Anteroposterior and lateral	Additional views if fat pad present
Shoulder	Anteroposterior and Y view	
Pelvis and sacrum	Anteroposterior only	Coccyx views rarely indicated
Hip	Anteroposterior and oblique	Anteroposterior of both hips and oblique or lateral of injured hip
Knee	Anteroposterior and lateral	Lateral is done with a horizontal beam
Ankle	Anteroposterior and lateral	Anteroposterior mortice view for trauma
Feet and toes	Anteroposterior and oblique	
Cervical spine	Anteroposterior, lateral, and peg	Lateral must show C7/T1 (otherwise computed tomography)
Thoracic spine and lumbar spine	Anteroposterior and lateral	
Chest	Posteroanterior erect or anteroposterior	Also anteroposterior supine (trauma)
Abdomen	Anteroposterior supine	Erect anteroposterior chest radiograph helpful
Head	Computed tomography scan	Plain skull radiographs rarely indicated
Face	Occipitomental and occipitomental 30°	Posteroanterior or posteroanterior 20°
Mandible	Anteroposterior view and orthopantomograph	Oblique view if orthopantomograph not available
Foreign bodies	Anteroposterior and lateral or tangential	Metal marker at entry site. Consider ultrasonography first or computed tomography

Rules of two

The rules of two are a simple set of guidelines. Most rules should be obvious and some relate to specific problems, but they are useful general principles that help to avoid errors in interpretation of radiographs and management of patients.

Rules of two

10 simple rules to follow
1 Two views: one view is one view too few
2 Two joints: image the joint above and below a long bone
3 Two sides: compare the other side (difficult cases only)
4 Two abnormalities: look for a second abnormality
5 Two occasions: compare current films with old films (especially for chest radiographs)
6 Two visits: repeat the film after a procedure or after an interval
7 Two opinions: ask colleague for opinion or use red dot system
8 Two records: write down clinical and radiographic findings
9 Two specialists: also get a formal radiological report
10 Two examinations: do not forget other tests such as ultrasonography, computed tomography, magnetic resonance imaging, and isotope bone scanning

1 Two views

Preferably, the two views should be perpendicular to each other. This rule applies to virtually all radiographs obtained, except for those of the chest, abdomen, and pelvis. Rarely, the abnormality is not visible at all or is subtle on the first view.

2 Two joints

Image the joint above and below a long bone. This particularly relates to mid-shaft injuries of the forearm (radius and ulna) and lower leg (tibia and fibula). Sometimes subtle injuries may be present in the joint above or below the obvious fracture.

3 Two sides

Rarely, the abnormality may be difficult to detect, and comparison with the other side can be helpful, especially in children. Always get a second opinion before requesting another radiograph because it means exposing the patient to additional radiation (an especially important consideration with children).

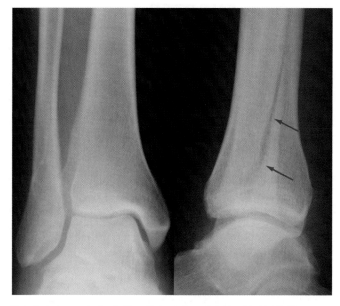

Rule 1 Anteroposterior (left) and lateral view of right ankle (right). The anteroposterior view was considered normal. The lateral view shows a displaced oblique fibula fracture (arrows).

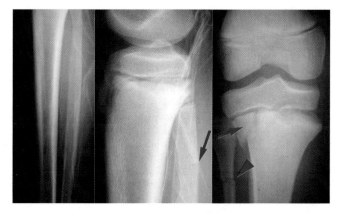

Rule 2 Anteroposterior view of right leg (left), lateral view of right knee (middle), and anteroposterior view of right knee (right). Shows a Salter-Harris type II injury – proximal tibial metaphysis is fractured, with separation and displacement of the epiphyseal growth plate and undisplaced fibula fracture (arrowhead).

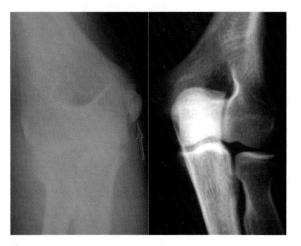

Rule 3 Anteroposterior view of right elbow (left) and anteroposterior view of left elbow (right). The right elbow has a non-united, avulsed, right medial epicondyle (arrow). The injury is obvious when compared with the normal left elbow with fused epiphyses.

4 Two abnormalities

Do not stop looking after you find one abnormality. An underlying predisposing cause may be the reason for the fracture (pathological fracture), or an unrelated incidental finding (such as a "bone island") might be present.

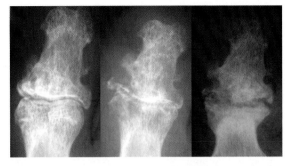

Rule 5 Septic arthritis in big toe. Initial film (left) was considered normal, but the loss of the joint space and the rapid progression confirms the diagnosis. The radiograph in the middle was taken when the diagnosis was made. The radiograph on the left was taken two weeks before, and the radiograph on the right was taken two weeks after the diagnosis.

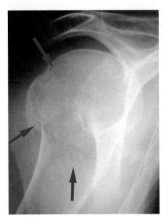

Rule 4 Anteroposterior view of right humerus shows pathological fracture through lytic metastasis (arrow).

5 Two occasions

If old films are available, always take the opportunity to look at them. This is particularly relevant in chest radiographs, because previous films will tell you if the latest radiograph shows an old or new finding. Similarly, if there is a bony abnormality, in particular if osteomyelitis or a septic arthritis is suspected, old films are essential for early diagnosis.

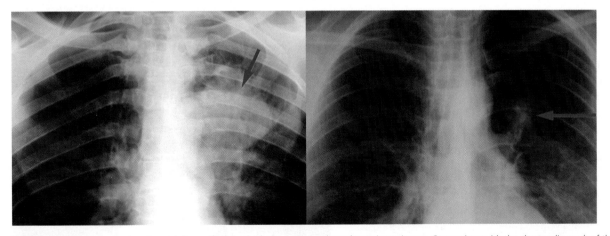

Rule 5 Posteroanterior chest radiograph (magnified view). Shows a primary bronchogenic carcinoma. Comparison with the chest radiograph of the same patient that was taken a year earlier (right) shows that the left hilar mass has enlarged over a year. The posteroanterior chest radiograph on the right (magnified view) was thought to be normal, but in retrospect, the tumour was visible (arrow).

6 Two visits

Always bring the patient back for a repeat set of radiographs after a procedure – especially after surgery, setting a fracture in plaster, reducing a dislocation, or removing a foreign body.

Sometimes the patient should come back for a repeat film after a set period of time to see whether the abnormality has resolved, got worse, or not changed. Classic scenarios in which this would be appropriate include a suspected scaphoid fracture or when abnormalities on chest radiographs are seen and an old film is not available for comparison.

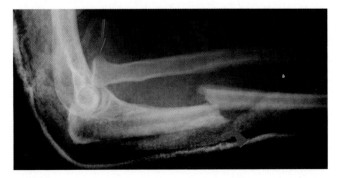

Rule 6 Lateral view of elbow in a plaster of Paris. Mid-shaft ulna is fractured (arrowhead), but the dislocated radial head had not been reduced (arrow).

7 Two opinions

Wherever possible, get a second opinion or show the radiograph to someone else. This is especially important if you are unsure about the radiograph. If the red dot system is used in your hospital, then this can be your first opinion.

The red dot system was introduced to help emergency department doctors. It is a voluntary system where the radiographer who took the radiograph gives his or her opinion as to whether the film is abnormal by placing a red dot next to the abnormality. It was initially, and in most hospitals still is, used for the peripheral skeleton only – that is, limb injuries. The red dot system helps to reduce errors and improve accuracy.

Radiographers are usually extremely experienced at taking films, looking at and interpreting them. Always ask the radiographer who took the film for their opinion first, especially if there is a red dot and you cannot find an abnormality.

8 Two records

Apart from recording the history and results of the examination, always record the findings of the radiograph. It is easy to look at the film and to forget to write down the findings. Films get lost, and your written record may be the only record.

9 Two specialists

All films should be seen and reported formally by a radiologist. This is particularly important for films that are at first thought to be normal because the patient is usually discharged and may not be seen by anyone else.

10 Two examinations

Sometimes, if the plain radiograph is normal, the symptoms may warrant further investigation. Studies have shown that if a scaphoid fracture is suspected and the scaphoid series of films are normal, the patient should have a magnetic resonance image scan when possible, rather than putting the patient in a splint or plaster and waiting 10-14 days before taking another set of films, which is "accepted normal management."

In addition, several abnormalities detected on plain radiographs warrant further imaging. If a fracture extends to the major joints (for example, acetabular and tibial plateau fractures), a computed tomography scan of the joint should be done routinely to evaluate the extent of joint involvement and to exclude loose fragments.

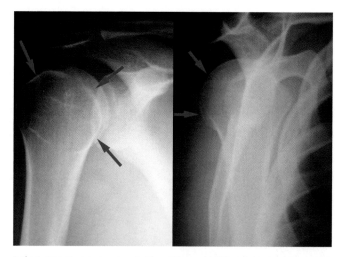

Rule 7 Anteroposterior view (left) and Y view (right) of right shoulder shows subtle posterior dislocation of the shoulder (arrow). Initially, these radiographs were interpreted as normal. The patient was then recalled to the emergency department by the radiologist for clinical review.

> **The more interesting a radiograph is, the more likely it will be stolen or lost**

> **The rules of two relate to what films to request, how to get help, and what to do next. This is an extension of the seventh commandment in Touquet's ten commandments of emergency radiology (see page 9)**

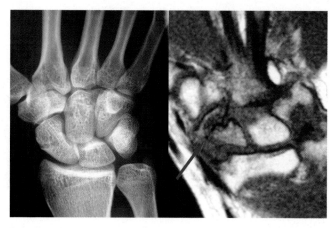

Rule 10 Anteroposterior view of scaphoid (left) and T1 weighted coronal magnetic resonance image (right) showing scaphoid fracture. Scaphoid series normal, but magnetic resonance image shows a fracture (arrow).

Ten commandments

Touquet's ten commandments are a simple set of guidelines to protect staff and hospitals from the inevitable mistakes that inexperienced doctors will make. Unfortunately, the commandments are often ignored. Many of the ten commandments are incorporated in the rules of two.

Command 1: treat the patient not the radiograph

Certain conditions or injuries should be treated on the basis of the clinical findings initially, especially if the injury is life threatening (such as a tension pneumothorax). With other injuries, delaying initial treatment to obtain a radiograph is unnecessary (for example, a dislocated ankle). The delay may be either life threatening, or have long term sequelae. In addition, a finding on the radiograph may be an incidental finding (the fourth rule in the rules of two).

> **Touquet's ten commandments of emergency radiology**
>
> - Command 1: treat the patient not the radiograph
> - Command 2: take a history and examine the patient before requesting a radiograph
> - Command 3: request a radiograph only when necessary
> - Command 4: never look at the radiograph without seeing the patient and never see the patient without reviewing the radiograph
> - Command 5: look at the radiograph, the whole radiograph and the radiograph as a whole in appropriate settings
> - Command 6: re-examine the patient when incongruity exists between the radiograph and the expected findings
> - Command 7: remember the rules of two
> - Command 8: take radiographs before and after procedures
> - Command 9: if a radiograph does not look quite right, ask and listen (the seventh rule of the rules of two)
> - Command 10: ensure you are protected by failsafe mechanisms

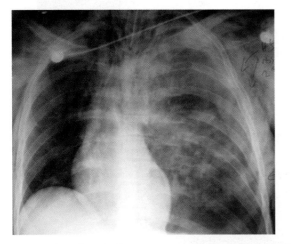

Command 1 Left tension haemopneumothorax. The patient should have been treated with a chest drain insertion before the chest radiograph was taken.

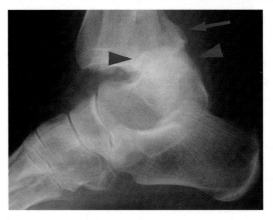

Command 1 Dislocated left ankle. The ankle should have been reduced without the radiograph.

> **Tension pneumothorax, dislocated joints (for example, hip or ankle), and a pulled elbow in a toddler are examples of conditions where treatment should be started on the basis of clinical findings**

Command 2: take a history and examine the patient before requesting a radiograph

A thorough clinical history and examination enables the mechanism of injury to be established, and the appropriate radiographs can then be requested. Knowledge of the mechanism of injury can often help to determine the likely pattern of injuries.

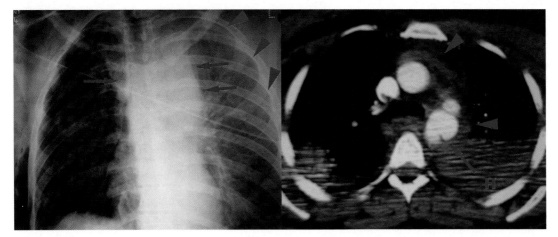

Command 2 Chest radiograph taken after a road crash (left) showing a widened mediastinum (arrow), and a haemothorax (arrowhead). A traumatic aortic injury was suspected and a computed tomogram was requested. The computed tomography image (right) confirms traumatic aortic injury (arrow) with associated mediastinal haematoma (arrowhead) and a large left haemothorax (H).

Command 3: request a radiograph only when necessary

Many requested investigations do not alter the patient's management, and in some cases they may be misleading. In head injuries, there is virtually no indication for performing a skull radiograph. Most patients who have sustained a substantial head injury should have a computed tomography scan. A safe approach to head injuries is always to scan it.

Command 4: never look at the radiograph without seeing the patient and never see the patient without reviewing the radiograph

Look at the radiograph properly, not be biased, and use a systematic approach. Always get the clinical history before giving an opinion. Then you will often pick up abnormalities that you may otherwise have missed. Never rely on someone else's opinion or report on radiographs if you have not seen the radiographs yourself. This is particularly relevant when patients are handed over at the end of a shift or when patients are transferred from elsewhere.

Command 5: look at the radiograph, the whole radiograph, and the radiograph as a whole in appropriate settings

In a pressured environment such as an emergency department, it is easy to rush and make mistakes. Interpreting radiographs too quickly inside a badly lit, noisy room with many distractions is a recipe for disaster. Interpretation of radiographs should be done in a calm manner in a quiet, well lit room using a viewing box or monitor. A common problem is that the person assessing the radiograph will focus immediately on expected abnormalities.

Even knowing the clinical history, try to ignore it at first and use a systematic approach. It is critical though that you always get the clinical history before giving your *final* opinion or report, because you must try to interpret the radiological findings in the context of the clinical presentation and answer the question.

Command 6: re-examine the patient when an incongruity exists between the radiograph and the expected findings

Review the radiographic findings in conjunction with the patient's history and your clinical findings. If the radiograph does not fit, review the history and clinical findings or ask for help. Many cases require further imaging – for example, request a magnetic resonance scan or an isotope bone scan in an elderly patient with a suspected fracture of the neck of femur, even if the initial plain radiographs seem normal.

Trauma to the coccyx, most clinically obvious nose fractures, head injuries (request a computed tomography scan), and simple rib fractures are examples of when radiographs are not necessary

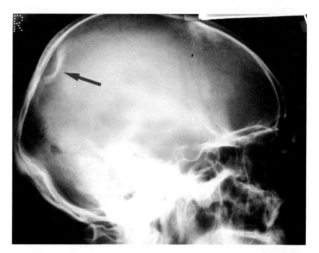

Command 3 Skull radiographs are not usually needed when dealing with head injuries. Important findings are generally subtle and often missed. This patient has a depressed skull fracture (arrow).

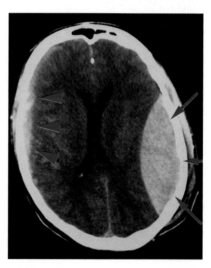

Command 3 Computed tomography image of head shows large left extradural haematoma (arrow) and subtle large right subdural haematoma (arrowhead).

In review clinics, radiographs are often lost or not available, but you must review previous radiographs. As a minimum, get the radiologist's report or repeat the films

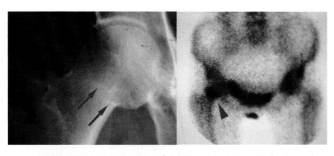

Command 6 Anteroposterior view of right hip showing subtle fracture of neck of femur (arrow), which was missed initially (left) and later confirmed on isotope bone scan as a fracture (arrowhead).

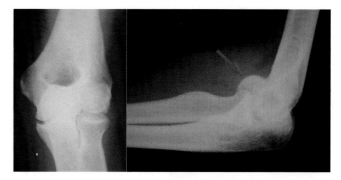

Command 6 Anteroposterior and lateral views of the elbow showing fracture-dislocation of capitellum. Patient clinically very tender with limited range of movement – review shows fracture and dislocation of capitellum (arrow).

Command 7: remember the rules of two

The original commandments included two views, two joints, two sides, and two occasions only (see the first, second, third, and fifth of the rules of two).

Command 8: take radiographs before and after procedures

See the sixth of the rules of two.

Command 9: if a radiograph does not look quite right, ask and listen

See the seventh of the rules of two.

Command 10: ensure you are protected by failsafe mechanisms

See the eighth and ninth of the rules of two. Abnormalities will be missed by all grades of staff and in all specialties. A report from a radiologist as well as personnel from the emergency staff, however, will minimise the effect of these errors on the patient and in the eyes of the law. Reports should be timely and accurate, and these failsafe mechanisms should be audited regularly. To miss an injury radiologically may not be negligent, but not to have a system in place to provide for this eventuality is negligent.

ABCs systematic assessment

The rules of two and the ten commandments are helpful guidelines for who, what, how, and when to radiograph and how to minimise the chances and consequences of errors.

The ABCs systematic assessment shows how to interpret radiographs. It is particularly helpful for junior doctors who have had little or no training on how to look at radiographs. This approach will help to familiarise them with the normal radiographs and minimise interpretive errors.

The ABCs systematic assessment is different for each type of body system. The ABCs for the peripheral skeleton are the same, but it is worth changing the order slightly to look for specific signs, in particular a fat pad sign in the elbow or a fat-fluid level (lipohaem-arthrosis) in the knee. Both of these signs are easy to detect and should alert you immediately to the presence of a probable fracture. Hence in the elbow and knee start by looking at soft tissues.

ABCs systematic assessment (the A also stands for anatomy in all systems)

Peripheral and axial skeleton
- **A**lignment
- **B**ones
- **C**artilage and joints
- **S**oft tissues and foreign bodies

Chest
- **A**dequacy, **a**ll lines and tubes and **a**irways – follow trachea and bronchi
- **B**reathing – Compare and contrast left and right lungs
- **C**irculation – Review heart, hila, and pulmonary vasculature
- **D**iaphragm
- **E**dges – Trace the pleura
- **S**keleton – Edge the bones, review **s**oft tissues, and seek foreign bodies

Abdomen
- **A**ir – Search for free intraperitoneal air and abnormal air
- **B**owel gas pattern
- **C**alcification
- **D**ensities – For example, look for foreign bodies, or tablets
- **E**dges – For example, hernial orifices, or lung bases
- **F**at planes – Relating to psoas, kidneys, and bladder
- **S**oft tissues and **s**keleton

Head (computed tomography scan)
- **A**irspaces
- **B**rains and bones
- **C**erebrospinal fluid spaces
- **D**ural spaces
- **E**yes
- **F**ace
- **S**oft tissues

Face
- **A**lignment – Trace McGrigor's and Campbell's lines
- **B**ones – Consider LeFort's classification
- **C**artilage – Delineate zygomaticofrontal suture and temporo-mandibular joints
- **D**ensities – Search for foreign bodies, glass, metal
- **S**oft tissues and sinuses – For example, frontal, ethmoid, and maxillary

Cervical spine (thoracic spine and lumbar spine)
- **A**dequacy, **a**ll lines and tubes, and **a**irway
- **A**lignment
- **B**ones
- **C**artilage – Check disc spaces and joints
- **S**oft tissues (prevertebral, paravertebral, and psoas)

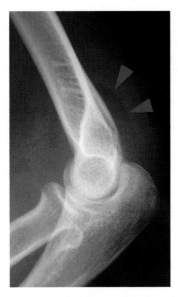

Lateral view of elbow – Look for fat pad sign first. An anterior (arrow) and posterior (arrowhead) fat pad sign indicate a probable fracture.

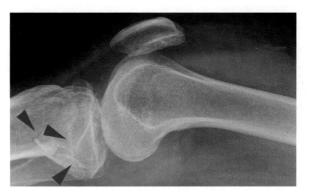

Horizontal beam lateral view of knee shows a lipohaemarthrosis (arrow). The fat (black) floats on the blood (white). This indicates a fracture (arrowhead), which in retrospect is visible.

KEY POINTS

- Request the correct radiographic examination
- Knowledge of anatomy is essential for evaluation of a radiograph
- Fundamental principles help reduce errors
- Remember the rules of two and the ten commandments
- Use a systematic approach to evaluate radiographs (ABCs)

Further reading

American College of Surgeons, Committee on Trauma. *Advanced trauma life support for doctors (ATLS) instructors' manual* Chicago: American College of Surgeons, 2005

Dick E, Francis I, Renfrew I. *Emergency radiology – rules and tools* London: Remedica, 2003

Keats TE. *Atlas of normal roentgen variants that may simulate disease.* St Louis: CV Mosby, 2001

Raby N, Berman L, de Lacey G. *Accident and emergency radiology: a survival guide.* 2nd ed. Philadelphia: Saunders, 2005

Rogers LF. *Radiology of skeletal trauma.* 3rd ed. London: Churchill Livingstone, 2004

Stern JE. *Trauma radiology companion.* Philadelphia: Lippincott, Williams and Wilkins, 1997

Touquet R, Driscoll P, Nicholson D. Teaching in accident and emergency medicine: 10 commandments of accident and emergency radiology. *BMJ* 1995;310:642-5

Touquet R, Fothergill J, Fertleman M, McCann P. Ten clinical safeguards for accident and emergency departments. *Clin Risk* 1999;1:44-9

Touquet R, Fothergill J, Henry J, Harris NH. Accident and emergency medicine. In Powers MJ, Harris NH, eds. *Clinical negligence.* 3rd ed. London: Butterworths, 2000

CHAPTER 2

Hand

Otto Chan, Tudor H Hughes

The hand is exposed and at risk of injury. It is therefore not surprising that hand injuries are the commonest skeletal injuries, and they account for 10-20% of attendances at accident and emergency departments. Fractures of the phalanges are more common than fractures of the metacarpals. Fractures of the distal phalanx account for half of all phalangeal fractures. Metacarpal injuries occur most commonly in the thumb and little finger.

Most injuries of the hands are easy to detect and correlate well with clinical findings. Identification of injuries is essential because early detection and appropriate management usually leads to recovery of normal function. Conversely, delay in diagnosis of what seems to be a minor abnormality can lead to a severe disability. Surgery is rarely necessary and only indicated for specific injuries. Clinical examination determines which radiographical views should be obtained.

Anatomy

Each finger consists of one metacarpal and three phalanges, and the thumb consists of one metacarpal and two phalanges. Each bone has a head, a shaft, and a base. Strong ulnar and radial collateral ligaments prevent sideways movement of the joints. The joint capsule of the interphalangeal and metacarpophalangeal joints is thickened on the palmar (volar) aspect and forms a dense fibrous structure (volar plate). This attaches to the base of the phalanx. Each finger has two flexor tendons and one extensor tendon. Sesamoid bones may be found on the palmar aspect of the hand, most commonly in the flexor tendons of the thumb at the level of the metacarpophalangeal joint.

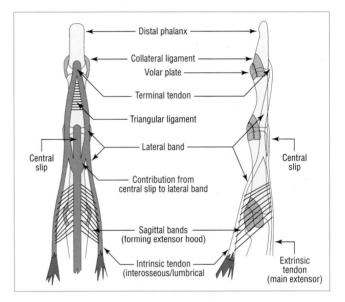

Dorsal (left) and lateral (right) view of left index finger.

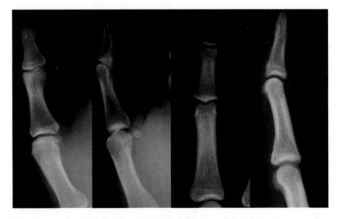

Anteroposterior (left) and lateral (middle left) view of thumb. Anteroposterior (middle right) and lateral (right) view of finger.

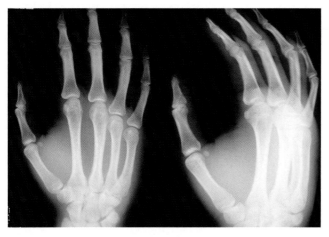

Anteroposterior (left) and oblique (right) view of the hand.

ABCs systematic assessment

Assessment of radiographs should follow the ABCs system:
- **A**dequacy and **a**lignment
- **B**one
- **C**artilage and joints
- **S**oft tissues.

Adequacy

Anteroposterior and lateral views should be obtained for finger injuries, and anteroposterior and oblique views are needed for hand injuries. Special views may be necessary for specific injuries, such as thumb injuries.

Alignment

Check the alignment of each finger and thumb on two views.

Bone

Exclude a fracture by carefully following the bony contour of each digit on two views. Then check the bone density and trabecular pattern. Occasionally, a vascular groove can be confused with a fracture.

Cartilage and joints

The joint space should be uniform in width. Overlap of bone margins may indicate a dislocation, and a second view should confirm this.

Soft tissues

Always use a bright light (or change the digital image windows) to look for soft tissue swelling. This may be the only sign of an injury. When radiographs are taken to detect foreign bodies a metallic marker should always be placed at the site of the injury, tangential to the site of entry. Foreign bodies may be visible on one view only.

Injuries

Distal phalanges
Crush fracture

This is an extremely common injury in which the tuft is squashed

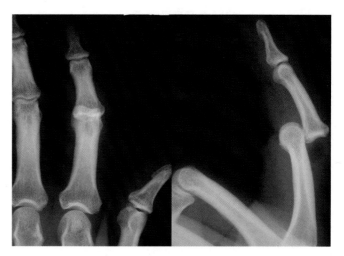

Anteroposterior (left) view of index finger showing soft tissue swelling over the proximal interpharangeal joint. The lateral view (right) confirms a dislocation.

ABCs systematic assessment

Adequacy and alignment
- Two views are needed to exclude dislocation of a finger
- Oblique or lateral view is needed to detect a Bennett's fracture
- Ultrasonography needed to detect gamekeeper's thumb

Bone
The commonest sites of injury are:
- Finger tip (crush fracture)
- Base of distal phalanx (mallet finger)
- Neck (base or shaft) of fifth metacarpal (boxer's fracture)

Cartilage and joints
- Look for overlapped joint space indicating subluxed or dislocated joint – for example, Bennett's fracture

Soft tissues
- A marker and a soft tissue exposure are needed for foreign body detection
- Radiography can localise soft tissue injury

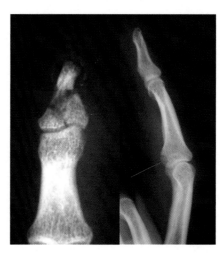

Anteroposterior view of index finger showing crush fracture (left) and volar plate avulsion (right).

and sustains a marginal chip or a comminuted fracture. Generally, a nail bed or pulp soft tissue injury is associated with a crush fracture.

Mallet finger (baseball finger)

Often caused by a direct blow to the extended digit—there is an avulsion of the extensor tendon at its insertion to the base of the distal phalanx. A less common injury is an avulsion of a small fragment of bone from the dorsal aspect of the base of the distal phalanx. The diagnosis is clinical and obvious—a flexion deformity of the distal interphalangeal joint.

Radiography is done to assess the size of the bony fragment. Most of these injuries heal with simple splinting of the joint (with a mallet splint), but complete tears of the tendon may need surgery.

Middle phalanges
Boutonnière deformity

This is a deformity of the digit with extension of the distal interphalangeal joint, flexion of the proximal interphalangeal joint, and no associated bony abnormality on the radiograph. The extensor mechanism attachment is torn, and splinting in hyperextension of the proximal interphalangeal joint is indicated to prevent a long term fixed flexion deformity.

Volar plate avulsion

This fracture is quite common. It is secondary to a hyperextension injury and sometimes associated with a dislocation of the proximal interphalangeal joint. The avulsed fragment of bone is often very small and difficult to identify. The fragment is sometimes seen only on an oblique view as a tiny flake of bone, and the clue to its presence is soft tissue swelling

Proximal phalanges
Spiral or transverse fracture

In this fracture the digit is often shortened and rotated; the injury is usually caused by of a direct blow. The deformity is generally more obvious when patients flex their fingers. Angulation is best evaluated with a true lateral view or oblique view. The anteroposterior view usually underestimates the degree of angulation and shortening.

Metacarpal bones
Punch fracture (boxer's fracture)

This is the direct result of a punch. The neck of the metacarpal is fractured, and there is volar displacement of the head. Usually the fifth metacarpal is damaged, but injury can also occur at the head of the fourth or other metacarpals. The history and clinical findings are characteristic (although patients often deny they have been in a fight) with flattening of the knuckle. A degree of angulation is accepted as this causes negligible functional disability.

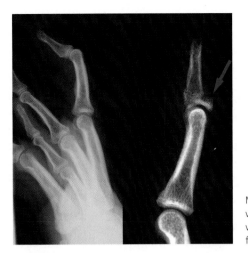

Mallet finger without (left) and with (right) avulsion fracture.

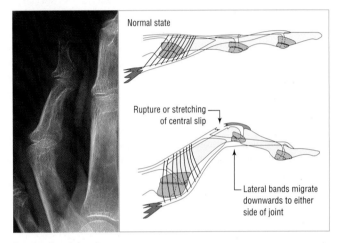

Boutonnière deformity.

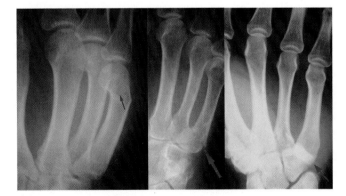

Punch fractures of fifth metacarpal – neck (left), base (middle), and fracture dislocation of the 4th and 5th carpometacarpal joints (right).

Other metacarpal injuries

Oblique or even transverse fractures of the shaft or base of the metacarpals and fracture and dislocation of the carpo metacarpal bones can occur. Sometimes the fracture occurs at the base and the carpometacarpal joint, and there is the possibility of an associated dislocation or subluxation of the joint. These fractures are sometimes best treated with pin fixation.

Thumb injuries
Bennett's fracture and dislocation

This is an oblique fracture of the base of the first metacarpal and dorsal dislocation or subluxation of the first metacarpal. The fracture extends to the carpometacarpal joint and the displacement is made worse and more unstable by the abductor muscles of the first metacarpal. The management of this injury is controversial. It can be treated by closed reduction with splinting, closed and percutaneous pin fixation, or open reduction and pinning. Referral to a specialist orthopaedic or hand surgeon is mandatory.

Gamekeeper's thumb (skier's thumb)

An abduction injury of the thumb occurs when there is outward distraction of the thumb and an avulsion of the attachment of the ulnar collateral ligament (which can be associated with a bony avulsion fracture). Stress films may show further widening of the joint space on the ulnar aspect, but these films are not recommended as they can aggravate the injury. Ultrasonography should confirm the diagnosis. These injuries may be treated conservatively, but complete tears of the ulnar collateral ligament may require surgery.

KEY POINTS

- History is important because the mechanism of injury often provides a clue to diagnosis
- Clinical examination will give a strong clue to the diagnosis
- Early diagnosis and appropriate management is essential for full recovery
- ABCs systematic approach should be used to review radiographs

---

We would like to thank Norbert Kang who kindly supplied the line drawings from which the figures of the dorsal and lateral views of the left index finger and the picture of the Boutonnière deformity were adapted.

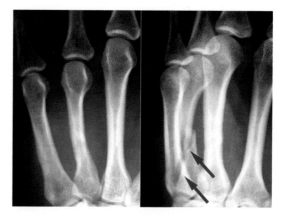

Anteroposterior view of the ring finger seems almost normal (left), but the oblique view shows an oblique fracture of shaft of fourth metacarpal (arrow).

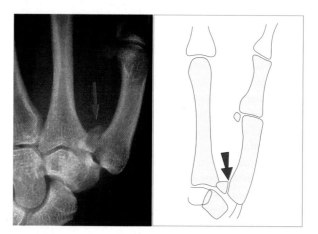

Bennett's fracture and dislocation of base of first metacarpal (arrow).

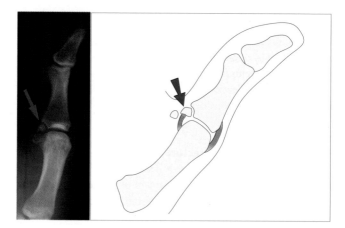

Gamekeeper's thumb (skier's thumb). Arrow shows fracture attached to ulnar collateral ligament (note the sesamoid).

CHAPTER 3

Wrist

Otto Chan, Caroline C Parlier-Cuau, Ali Naraghi

Fractures of the distal forearm and wrist are the most common skeletal injuries, and most are the result of a fall onto an outstretched hand. The mechanisms of injury are similar, and the resultant injury depends on several factors. Age alone, however, is a good predictor of the likely injury. Carpal bones are rarely injured in children. Children younger than 10 years will probably sustain a metaphyseal transverse fracture, and those aged 11-16 years sustain injuries through the epiphyseal growth plate (Salter-Harris fractures). People aged 17-40 years tend to sustain scaphoid and avulsion triquetral fractures. Older patients (more than 60 years) with osteoporotic bones sustain Colles' fractures of the distal radius and ulna. In a Colles' fracture, the distal radius fracture is displaced onto the dorsal aspect of the wrist. Rarely (but of importance), the distal radius component is displaced onto the palmar aspect (Smith's fracture) or fracture dislocation of the radiocarpal bones (Barton's fracture) occurs.

Occasionally, a single fracture of the shaft of the radius is associated with a dislocation of the distal radioulnar joint (Galeazzi's fracture). The reverse of Galeazzi's fracture is a single fracture of the ulna, with associated dislocation of the radial head in the elbow (Monteggia fracture). Dislocation of the carpal bones usually involves the lunate; other carpal dislocations are extremely rare.

Unfortunately, many wrist fractures and dislocations can be subtle or initially seem normal on radiography (beware of scaphoid fracture), and clinical findings may be minimal.

> **Identification of injuries to the wrists (such as injuries to the hands) is essential, because early detection and appropriate management usually leads to recovery of normal function. Conversely, delay in diagnosis of even the most seemingly minor abnormality (for example, a scaphoid fracture) can lead to severe disability and long term problems**

> **Factors that affect injuries of forearm and wrist**
>
> - Age of patient
> - Severity of injury
> - Direction of force
> - Angle and position of joints at maximum impact

Age related injuries

Age (years)	Type of injury
4-10	Torus and greenstick fractures
11-16	Salter-Harris injuries
17-40	Scaphoid and triquetral fractures
>60	Colles' fractures

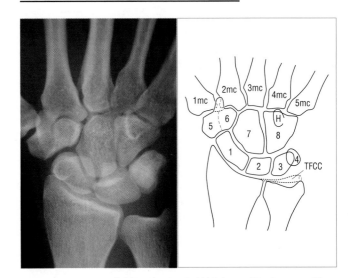

Anteroposterior view of right wrist. Scaphoid (1), lunate (2), triquetrum (3), pisiform (4), trapezium (5), trapezoid (6), capitate (7), hamate (8). (H=hook of hamate, mc=metacarpal, TFCC=triangular fibrocartilage complex).

Anatomy

The wrist contains two rows of carpal bones.
- The proximal row articulates with the distal radius and ulna and the triangular fibrocartilage complex
- The distal row articulates with the base of the metacarpals (carpometacarpal joint).

The carpal bones are held together by strong intercarpal ligaments (for example, the scapho-lunate and lunate-triquetral ligaments). The distal radius is held to the ulna by the triangular fibrocartilage complex, which inserts to the base of the ulnar styloid.

The carpal joint has a 10-15° volar or palmar angulation. In addition, the radial styloid is distal to the ulnar styloid, so the hand is usually held in slight ulnar deviation and slight flexion (hold your hand out to see this).

A square muscle, the pronator quadratus, lies flat on the volar (palmar) aspect of the distal radius and ulna. This can be identified as a fat plane on almost all radiographs. Displacement, bowing, or loss of this fat plane suggests the presence of a distal radius fracture. The fat plane is of more relevance, however, because a completely normal fat plane for the pronator quadratus virtually rules out a serious fracture.

The carpal bones in children (primary ossification centres) first appear at about the age of three months (capitate), and all the carpal bones are visible by six years. The age of the child at this time can be estimated by counting the number of epiphyses visible minus one. Secondary ossification centres (epiphyses) of the metacarpals and phalanges appear at the age of 2-3 years and fuse by puberty. Hand radiographs can be used to assess the bone age of a child up to the age of 18 years.

ABCs systematic assessment

- Adequacy
- Alignment
- Bone
- Cartilage and joints
- Soft tissues

Adequacy

Anteroposterior and lateral views should be obtained for wrist injuries. If a scaphoid fracture is suspected, a scaphoid series should be obtained (four coned views).

Alignment
Anteroposterior view

Look at the anteroposterior view first. Check that all the joint spaces are the same (1-2 mm) and parallel in an adult. Draw lines through the top and bottom of the scaphoid, lunate, and triquetrum. Then draw a third line through the proximal surface of the distal carpal bones. Disruption of these parallel lines (Gilula's arcs) may suggest carpal instability or a subluxation or dislocation of a carpal bone. The pisiform is superimposed on the triquetrum.

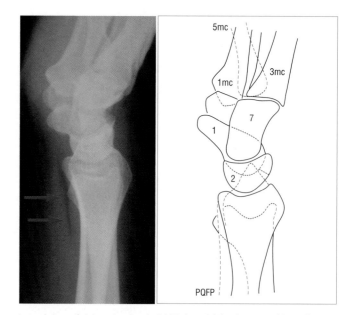

Lateral view of right wrist. Scaphoid (1), lunate (2), triquetrum (3), pisiform (4), trapezium (5), trapezoid (6), capiate (7), hamate (8). (mc=metacarpal, PQFP=pronator quadratus fat pad).

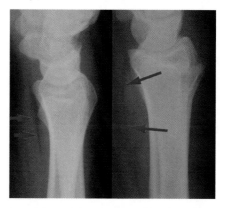

Lateral views of the wrist. Normal fat plane of pronator quadratus (arrows in left radiograph), displaced fat plane of pronator quadratus (arrows in right radiograph).

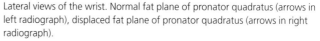

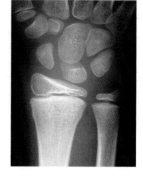

Anterior view of right wrist showing the three parallel arcs.

Normal anteroposterior view of hand in a child aged six years.

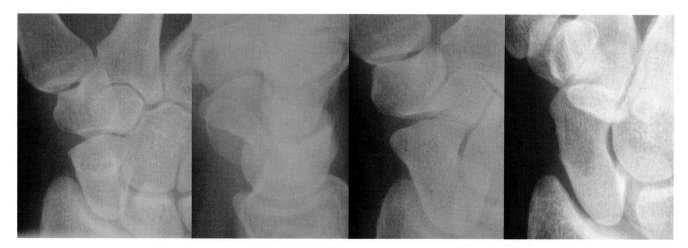

Scaphoid views – anteroposterior (left), lateral (middle left), oblique view (middle right), and dedicated scaphoid view (right).

Check the lunate has a square appearance (a triangular shape indicates a lunate or perilunate dislocation). Widening of the joint space of the scaphoid and lunate indicates a scapholunate joint disruption, and a tear of the scapholunate ligament.

The distal ulna should overlap slightly the distal radius or almost touch it; separation suggests distal radioulnar joint disruption. The distal radius should be distal to the distal ulnar styloid with a 5-10° ulnar deviation (if not, suspect a distal radius fracture [Colles' fracture] or a dislocation of the ulna).

Lateral view

The lateral view is the key to not missing an important injury. The radius, lunate, capitate, and base of the third metacarpal all should articulate with each other. The lunate should look like a moon (hence lunate), and its concavity always should face distally and be filled by the capitate. If the lunate concavity is empty, a lunate or perilunate dislocation is present. The palmar angulation of the radiocarpal joint should be 10-15°.

Bone

Anteroposterior view

Check the overall contour and bony margins of each bone and then the trabecular pattern – starting proximally and working distally. Look particularly for a linear lucency, for a line of sclerosis (a white line that indicates an impacted fracture), or for a cortical break.

Lateral view

This is often the only view that shows an abnormality, particularly subtle distal radius fractures, carpal dislocations, and triquetral fractures. Any flake of bone lying in the dorsal aspect of the carpal bones probably represents an avulsion fracture of the triquetrum.

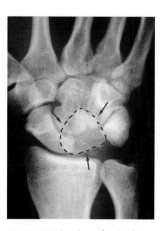

Anteroposterior view of wrist shows triangular lunate (arrows) consistent with a lunate dislocation.

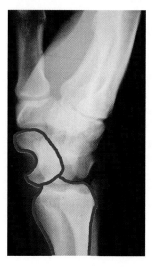

Lateral view of wrist shows dislocated lunate.

Cartilage and joints

The importance of checking that all joint spaces are the same cannot be emphasised enough. Narrowing of a joint space can be caused by technical factors (such as rotation) or disease (such as osteoarthritis). An increase in the joint space may indicate carpal instability, particularly of the scapholunate joint.

Soft tissues

Look for soft tissue swelling. This will often indicate the site of injury. Check that the fat pad of the pronator quadratrus is intact and is not displaced.

The fat stripe of the scaphoid is a radiolucency that lies on the radial side of the scaphoid. This was thought to be helpful in the diagnosis of a scaphoid fracture. Unfortunately, this sign is not usually seen in children younger than 12 years, and so is unreliable.

Injuries

Distal radius and ulna

Torus fracture – A buckle of the cortex from a longitudinal compression injury in a child. This usually occurs in the distal radius and is not associated with any substantial displacement. Torus fractures can be subtle and are often seen only on one view.

Greenstick fracture – A fracture with complete disruption on one side of the cortex but continuity of the cortex on the other side from an angular force. The torus fracture usually occurs at the radius, but the greenstick fracture also may involve the ulna. This fracture is often associated with a slight deformity and is usually easy to detect.

Salter-Harris fracture – An injury of the epiphysis and epiphyseal growth plate of children that is predominantly seen in children aged 11-16 years. Injuries to the wrist account for up to half of all Salter-Harris injuries. A fall onto an outstretched hand leads to a shearing injury into the growth plate, which usually results in a Salter-Harris type II injury. Salter-Harris classification is discussed in Chapter 16.

Colles' fracture – A common injury in middle aged people and particularly in older patients. The distal radius is fractured, with evidence of dorsal angulation on the lateral view. Some shortening of the distal radius usually occurs, and, as a consequence of this, associated radial deviation of the hand and wrist are seen. An associated fracture of the ulnar styloid often occurs; this is of no important clinical consequence. Rarely, however, an associated scaphoid fracture can occur; this should not be overlooked because it has serious consequences.

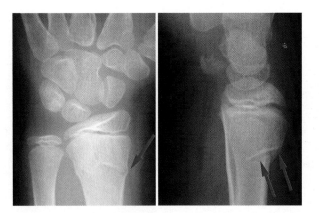

Torus fracture – anteroposterior view shows only a bump (arrow in left radiograph); the buckle is better seen on the lateral view (arrows on right radiograph).

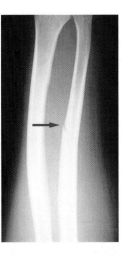

Greenstick fracture – mid-shaft ulna. Anteroposterior view of the forearm in a child.

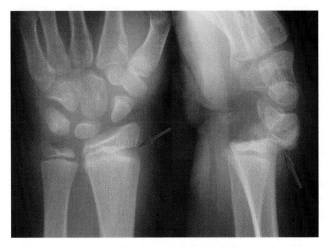

Salter-Harris type I injury with a fracture of the epiphysis (arrows): anteroposterior view (left), lateral view (right radiograph).

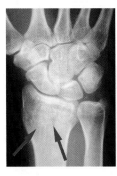
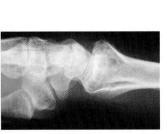

Colles' fracture.

Smith's fracture – A rare injury in which the distal radius fracture has a palmar angulation. This fracture is the opposite of a Colles' fracture and should be referred to an orthopaedic surgeon.

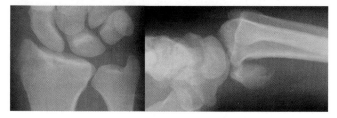

Smith's fracture.

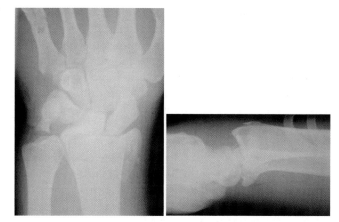

Barton's fracture.

Barton's fracture – A fracture dislocation of the radiocarpal joint. The fracture of the distal radius extends to the joint surface, with palmar or dorsal displacement of the carpal bones.

Galeazzi's fracture-dislocation – A fracture of the distal radius shaft with associated shortening of the radius. As a result, disruption of the distal radio-ulnar joint occurs. On radiographs, the ulna will look too long, with associated radial deviation of the wrist and hand.

Monteggia fracture-dislocation – The reverse of a Galeazzi's fracture. A fracture of the ulna (often proximal or mid-shaft) occurs, with associated shortening, and therefore disruption, of the radio-capitelar joint. Radiographs show dislocation of the radial head at the elbow joint.

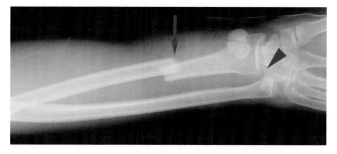

Galeazzi's fracture. The forearm radiograph shows the radial fracture (arrow) and dislocation at the distal radioulnar joint (arrowhead).

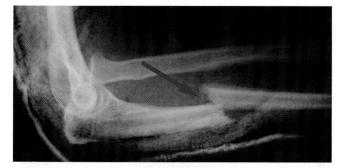

Monteggia fracture in plaster of Paris showing a fracture of the mid-ulna (arrow) and dislocation of the radial head (arrowhead).

Carpal bones

Scaphoid fracture – The most common carpal bone to fracture (> 90%). The fractures are usually displaced only minimally and, therefore, are often subtle or not visible at all on the initial radiographic views. Correct diagnosis and management of these injuries are needed to avoid the late complications of non-union or avascular necrosis. A four view series is obtained, and, even if no fracture is seen, the patient should be treated initially as if they have a scaphoid fracture. Alternatively, further imaging with an isotope study or magnetic resonance imaging should be done to exclude an injury. The presence or absence of a scaphoid fat pad is not a helpful sign.

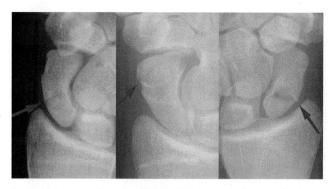

Scaphoid views showing acute fractures of the waist (left), proximal pole (middle) of the scaphoid, as well as an older fracture (right).

Blood supply, which runs distal to proximal, can be compromised to the proximal portion of the fracture. This leads to delayed union, which in turn can cause non-union or avascular necrosis. The vascular supply to the proximal segment of the waist of the scaphoid fractures therefore may be compromised; it is always compromised in proximal pole fractures. Distal pole fractures usually heal well. Most of the fractures occur at the waist (>70%); the remainder are proximal (20%) or distal (10%).

Other carpal bone fractures – The triquetrum is the second most common fracture of the carpal bones and represents an avulsion flake fracture seen only on the lateral view, which usually heals. Other carpal bone fractures are unusual, and, even if present, they are rarely detected on plain radiographs.

Carpal dislocations are uncommon and invariably involve the lunate. The key to detecting these injuries lies in the anatomy of the lunate and its relation to the other surrounding carpal bones; an understanding of the lateral view is particularly helpful. On the anteroposterior view, the joint space of all the carpal bones should be the same (1-2 mm), and the lunate should have a "square" appearance. Note the alignment of the distal radius, lunate, capitate, and base of the third metacarpal on the anteroposterior and lateral views. The lunate should always articulate with the capitate, and the concavity of the lunate should face upwards and be filled by the capitate.

In lunate dislocations, the lunate on the anteroposterior view often looks triangular, and the joint space is usually widened, particularly with the scaphoid. On the lateral view, the lunate concavity faces forward (palmar) and is empty. Alignment of the radius, capitate, and third metacarpal is maintained.

Perilunate dislocations are less common and are often accompanied by other injuries, particularly scaphoid fractures. The appearance of the anteroposterior view is similar to that for a lunate dislocation, but on the lateral view, the empty lunate concavity faces upwards. The distal radius and lunate are aligned, and, similarly, the capitate and base of the third metacarpal are aligned, but the capitate lies behind (dorsal to) the lunate.

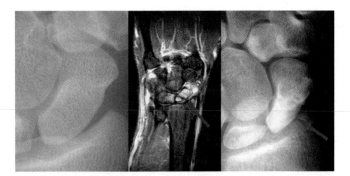

Scaphoid: normal posteroanterior radiograph (left), magnetic resonance image (T2 weighted fat suppressed sequence) showing oedema of the scaphoid with a proximal pole fracture (arrow), and posteroanterior radiograph showing avascular necrosis of the scaphoid (arrow in right radiograph).

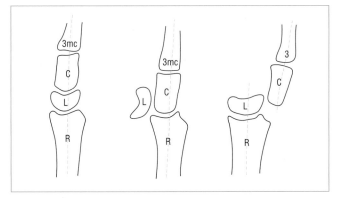

Lateral wrist: normal (left), lunate dislocation (middle), and perilunate dislocation (right). (C=capitate L=lunate, mc=metacarpal, R=radius).

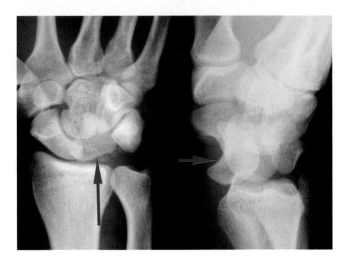

Lunate dislocation.

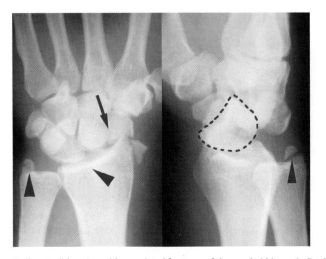

Perilunate dislocation with associated fractures of the scaphoid (arrow), distal radius and ulna (arrowhead).

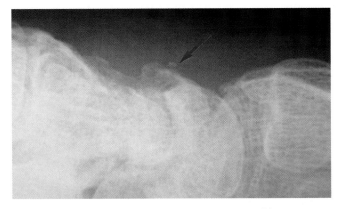

Magnified lateral radiograph of the wrist showing a triquetral fracture.

KEY POINTS

- Diagnosis should be made on the basis of clinical examination
- If scaphoid tenderness is present four views should be requested, and the patient should be treated as if they have a scaphoid fracture
- The lunate anatomy should be reviewed to exclude a dislocation or carpal instability
- Dorsal bony fragments represent avulsion triquetral fracture.
- Early diagnosis and appropriate management are essential for full recovery

ABCs systematic assessment

Alignment

- An intercarpal joint space exceeding 2-3 mm indicates carpal instability
- Disruption of the arcs indicates carpal instability
- Radial styloid should be distal to the ulnar styloid – otherwise suspect Colles' fracture

Bone

- A buckled cortex indicates a torus fracture
- Dorsally angulated radius indicates a Colles' fracture
- Palmar angulated radius indicates a Smith's fracture
- Triangular lunate on an anteroposterior radiograph indicates a carpal dislocation
- An empty lunate concavity on the lateral view indicates carpal dislocation
- If there is tenderness of the scaphoid but the radiographs look normal treat as scaphoid fracture; repeat radiographs at two weeks or consider magnetic resonance imaging
- Bone flake on the dorsal aspect of the carpus on a lateral view indicates a triquetral avulsion fracture

Cartilage and joints

- Widened joint space indicates carpal instability

Soft tissues

- A displaced fat pad of the pronator quadratus indicates a distal radius fracture

CHAPTER 4

Elbow

Gerald de Lacey, Otto Chan

Elbow injuries are common and usually result from a fall onto an outstretched hand. Detecting and interpreting abnormal features on radiographs can be difficult and challenging – particularly in children because they have multiple epiphyseal and apophyseal growth centres. An understanding of normal anatomy and adoption of a systematic approach when assessing the radiographs are essential.

The elbow joint

- Three articulations
  - Humero-ulnar
  - Humero-radial
  - Radio-ulnar
- A single synovial lining
- A layer of shock absorbent fat between the synovium and capsule
- Three strong ligaments
  - Ulnar collateral
  - Radial collateral
  - Annular

Anatomy

The elbow is a hinge joint that consists of three articulations within a single synovial space. The lower end of the humerus is composed of two different shapes. On the lateral side, a partly spherical contour (capitellum) articulates with the concave articular surface of the head of the radius. On the medial side, a notched medial contour (trochlea) articulates with the ulna.

The stability of the radio-ulnar articulation is maintained by the annular ligament. In effect, this is a sling that holds the head of the radius against the ulna. The radial head is free to rotate within this sling.

The joint capsule comprises an inner layer of synovium, a layer of fat, and an outer layer of fibrous tissue. The layer of fat results in anterior and posterior fat pads. These lie outside the synovial lining of the joint, but within the joint capsule. The anterior fat pad is radiographically visible in almost all normal elbows. The posterior fat pad lies deep in the olecranon fossa and is never visible in the flexed position unless a large effusion or haemarthrosis displaces it out of the fossa.

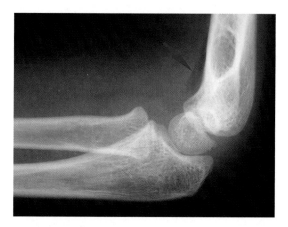

Normal anterior fat pad (arrow) lies adjacent to the cortex of the humerus. Note that the posterior fat pad is not seen in the normal flexed elbow – it is hidden deep in the olecranon fossa. (The supinator fat stripe is seen as a horizontal black line parallel to the anterior aspect of the radial shaft. Its appearance is sometimes claimed to be useful in terms of diagnosis, but in practice it is best to ignore it.)

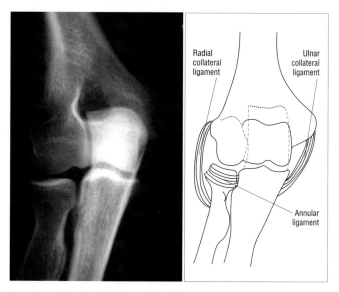

Anteroposterior view of elbow and line drawing showing ligaments. The annular ligament is wrapped around four fifths of the head of the radius.

Descriptive terms

- Internal epicondyle – medial epicondyle
- External epicondyle – lateral epicondyle
- Capitellum – capitulum
- Epiphysis – growing part at the end of a long bone. It is separated from the shaft of the bone by a layer of cartilage
- Apophysis – secondary ossification centre that does not form part of a joint surface. It produces a protrusion or tubercle and contributes to the final shape of the bone. Usually the site of attachment of a tendon or ligament. Until the apophysis fuses to the main bone, it is separated from the bone by a layer of cartilage
- Monteggia fracture dislocation (or lesion) – fracture of the ulna with an associated dislocation of the head of the radius
- Pulled elbow – nursemaid's elbow

Children

Because a child's elbow has unfused ossification centres it is more vulnerable to a particular set of injuries than is an adult's elbow. Children have three epiphyseal ossification centres (capitellum, trochlea, and radius) and three apophyseal centres (internal epicondyle, external epicondyle, and olecranon). These begin to ossify at different ages. The trochlear and olecranon centres are often multicentric. This multicentric appearance should not be mistaken for fracture fragments. If the appearance is confusing, refer to a textbook of normal variants or seek a specialist opinion. Very occasionally it is necessary to radiograph the opposite uninjured elbow to make a comparison.

The acronym CRITOE (capitellum, radial head, internal epicondyle, trochlea, olecranon, external epicondyle) lists the most common sequence in which the secondary ossification centres appear on the radiograph. Although the CRITOE order is the most common sequence, individual variation in the CRITOE procession does occur. Nevertheless, one part of the sequence never varies: the internal epicondyle always ossifies before the trochlea. This has particular diagnostic relevance to an uncommon, but clinically important, injury involving major displacement of the internal epicondyle ossification centre.

ABCs systematic assessment

- Adequacy
- Alignment
- Bones
- Congruity
- Soft tissues

Adequacy

There are two standard radiographic projections: anteroposterior and lateral. A severe injury will often make perfect positioning impossible. Other additional projections are sometimes provided in order to show the head and neck of the radius to better advantage. These extra views are not routine and are generally requested for specific reasons only.

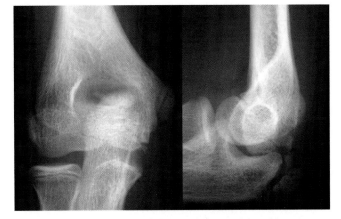

Normal appearance in a boy aged 13 years. All the ossification centres are present. The trochlear and olecranon secondary centres are multicentric. These multiple centres are common normal variants.

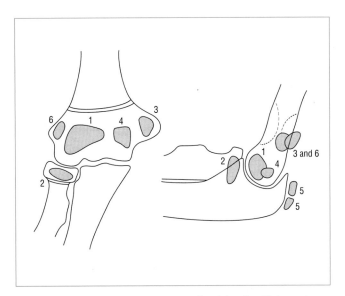

Normal secondary ossification centres: capitellum (1), radius (2), internal epicondyle (3), trochlea (4), olecranon (5), and external epicondyle (6). Note: on the lateral projection, the centre for the internal or external epicondyle may be seen surprisingly far posterior – this is normal. Also, the olecranon is multicentric – this is normal.

Approximate age at which secondary ossification centres appear on radiographs (CRITOE)

Centre	Appears	Age (years)
Capitellum	First	12 months
Radial head	Second	3-6
Internal epicondyle	Third	4-7
always before the …		
Trochlea	Fourth	7-10
Olecranon	Fifth	6-10
External epicondyle	Sixth	11-14

NB The sequence in which the secondary centres appear (above) is the most common sequence. There are occasional individual variations.

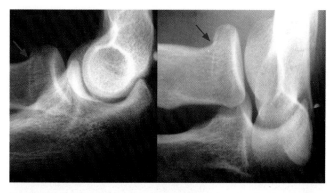

Standard lateral projection and an angled view to show head and neck of the radius. In this patient, the subtle cortical break at the junction of the head and neck is shown well. The white line that crosses the neck of the radius is caused by slight impaction.

Alignment

Lateral radiograph

The olecranon articulates with the trochlea, and the radial head articulates with the capitellum. Note that the trochlea and capitellum are superimposed on each other on the lateral view. Two lines need to be assessed on the lateral view.

Radio-capitellar line – The shaft of a normal radius, as seen on the lateral projection, is not always a perfectly straight line. Its proximal 2-4 cm may be set at an angle to the long axis of the rest of the bone. A line drawn along the centre of the long axis of this proximal 2-4 cm of the radius should pass through the capitellum. If this line passes behind or in front of the capitellum, then a dislocated head of the radius is present.

Anterior humeral line – There is a range of normal condylar shapes. Nevertheless, all normal elbows show a hockey stick or J shaped contour. Loss of the hockey stick contour suggests a displaced supracondylar fracture.

A line drawn along the anterior cortex of the humerus should have a third or more of the blade of the hockey stick (that is, the capitellum) lying anterior to it. If this rule is broken, there will probably be a supracondylar fracture with posterior displacement of the distal fragment. The anterior humeral line is also useful to assess the degree of posterior displacement when a fracture is obvious.

> The rule relating to the anterior humeral line does not apply in a very young child with a normal elbow because the amount of ossification in the capitellum is not yet large enough to have a third in front of the anterior cortex of the humerus

X sign or hour glass sign – This can be helpful in the diagnosis of a supracondylar fracture. The X appearance (which can be likened to an hour glass) is made up of the bone margins of the olecranon and the coronoid fossae. A supracondylar fracture almost always disrupts the normal X on a true lateral radiograph.

Anteroposterior radiograph

The radio-capitellar and coronoid-trochlear joint spaces should be parallel and spaced equally. In normal adults, and in most children, a line drawn along the centre of the long axis of the radius (note: along

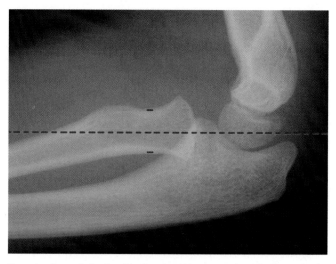

Normal radio-capitellar line. The line should be drawn along the long axis of the proximal 2-4 cm of the radius. This part of the radius is often angled in relation to the rest of the shaft. If the line was drawn along the long axis of the distal two thirds of the radius then (in many normal people) it would not pass through the capitellum; an erroneous diagnosis of a dislocated head of radius would then be made.

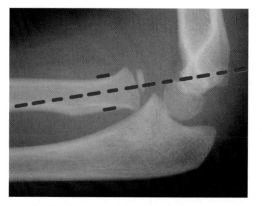

Dislocated head of radius. The radio-capitellar line does not pass through the centre of the capitellum. (Incidentally, note the normal X or hour glass appearance superimposed on the shaft of the humerus).

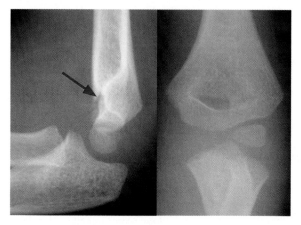

A girl aged three years fell on an outstretched hand. The radio-capitellar line is normal. The anterior humeral line does not pass through the middle third of the capitellum, and the normal X appearance is disrupted. This is a supracondylar fracture with posterior displacement. The fracture is visible on the lateral projection, but it is barely detectable on the anteroposterior view.

the proximal 2-4 cm) will pass through the capitellum. If it does not do so then the lateral radiograph should be checked for evidence of a dislocation of the head of the radius.

> In a young child with a normal elbow, the rule above does not apply if the forearm is rotated slightly

Bones
Lateral radiograph
Examine the cortical surfaces of the humerus, radius, and ulna. A subtle break in the anterior humerus from a supracondylar fracture can be hard to detect, especially in a child. Check the X appearance (made up of the deep bone margins of the olecranon and coronoid fossae). A disrupted X appearance is indicative of a supracondylar fracture.

Examine the internal trabecular pattern of the bones for bands of increased density. An impacted radial neck fracture may be visible only as a faint transverse band of increased density at the junction of the head and the neck. Bruising or damage to cartilage does occur, but it will not show on a radiograph.

Anteroposterior radiograph
About half of all radial head fractures are undisplaced, and a radiographic abnormality can be subtle. Slight cortical disruption, faint depression, and/or slight angulation should be looked for. In addition, in children:

- Check for a faint lucent line crossing the distal humerus – this is often the only evidence of either an undisplaced supracondylar fracture or a fracture of the lateral condyle of the humerus.
- Check that the medical epicondyle is in a normal position. Specifically, make sure that it is not trapped in the joint and masquerading as a trochlear ossification centre. This is a rare injury. Children with a dislocation of the elbow joint that reduces spontaneously are the group most at risk.

If the medial epicondyle is trapped within the joint, minor but detectable widening of the medial part of the joint will occur. Consequently, the joint's normal congruity is altered. The trapped epicondyle is rarely seen on an anteroposterior projection – it will be seen more clearly on a lateral radiograph.

> Fractures of the lateral epicondyle account for 20% of elbow fractures in children

Congruity
Congruity of articular surfaces should be confirmed:
- The trochlea is congruous with the ulna
- The capitellum is congruous with or parallels the articular surface of the radial head

Loss of congruity or parallelism will be seen with some radial head fractures.

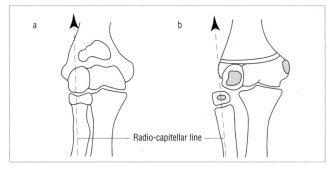

The radio-capitellar line also applies to the anteroposterior projection – with a caveat. The line is drawn along the central axis of the proximal 2-4 cm of the radius and it should pass through the capitellum (a). If it does not, suspect a dislocated head of the radius. The caveat: in very young children, a slightly rotated forearm can cause the rule to be invalidated and lead to a false-positive diagnosis of dislocation (b). Be safe … always correlate the anteroposterior appearance with the more reliable position of the radio-capitellar line on the lateral projection.

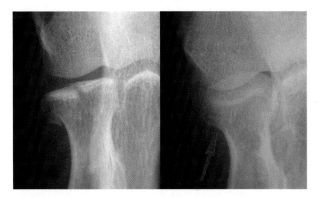

Fracture of the head and neck of the radius (left): this slightly impacted intra-articular fracture is obvious. The fracture shown on the right is much more subtle: a faint lucent line crosses the articular surface and a minute break in the lateral cortex of the neck (arrow) is also present.

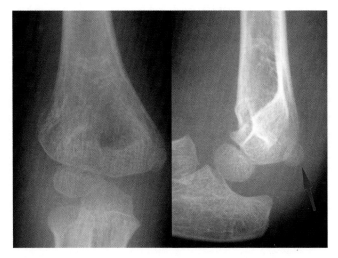

The lack of definition and slight disruption of the cortex of the humerus indicates an undisplaced fracture of the lateral condyle. The posterior fat pad is visible indicating a large haemarthrosis. Incidentally, note that the ossification centre for the internal epicondyle is situated far posteriorly on the lateral radiograph – this is normal (arrow).

Soft tissues

Lateral radiograph

The normal anterior fat pad appears as a thin elongated radiolucency lying parallel and adjacent to the distal cortex of the humerus. A posterior fat pad is not identified in a normal elbow held in flexion. Displacement of these fat pads occurs when there is an intra-articular effusion (for example, a haemarthrosis) displacing the synovial lining.

- A displaced anterior fat pad appears as a triangular shaped black lucency anterior to the cortex of the humerus – but elevated off the bone. Sometimes this displacement is referred to as the sail sign.
- The posterior fat pad requires a large effusion to push it out of the deep olecranon fossa. It is then visualised as a black line just posterior to the cortex of the humerus.
- The rules to apply:
  – positive anterior fat pad sign: an effusion is present… an intra-articular fracture is likely
  – positive posterior fat pad sign: a very large effusion is present… an intra-articular fracture is even more likely.

Note: Some authors refer to a supinator fat stripe. Claims that the appearance of this lucent line is helpful in diagnosing a bone injury have been shown to be over optimistic. The supinator fat stripe can be ignored.

Lateral radiograph – soft tissue rules

- Positive anterior fat pad sign: an effusion is present … a fracture is likely
- Positive posterior fat pad sign: a large effusion is present …a fracture is highly likely
- Absence of a fat pad sign: does not mean "no fracture"

Anteroposterior radiograph

If an injury has occurred to the medial or lateral epicondyes, adjacent soft tissue swelling will be present.

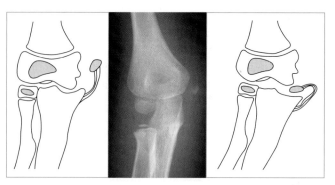

Moderate avulsion of the internal epicondyle secondary centre (left and middle). Major avulsion of the epicondyle (right): it lies within the joint and can be misinterpreted as a trochlear ossification centre. The internal epicondyle always ossifies before the trochlea so suspect that an internal epicondyle lies in the joint if it is not seen in its normal position. Often, when the epicondyle is trapped in the joint there is a slight widening of the medial part of the joint on the anteroposterior projection.

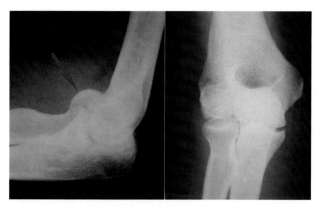

There is an additional rounded bone fragment seen on the lateral, which should not be there (arrow) and represents a fracture – dislocation of the capitellum. The anteroposterior radiograph looks almost normal but careful inspection of the capitellum confirms a subtle fracture.

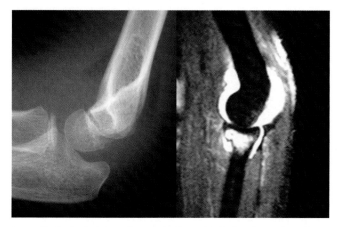

Large effusion in the joint – the anterior fat pad is displaced away from the cortex of the humerus and the posterior fat pad is visible. No fracture shown (left). Magnetic resonance image – sagittal FST2 shows joint effusion with radial head fracture (right). The message: a large effusion on the radiograph makes a fracture highly probable; probable but not certain.

Other injuries

The radius and ulna are bound together by the strong interosseous ligament. If one of the forearm bones sustains a displaced or angulated fracture, the other bone will invariably fracture. If this additional fracture is not seen then look for:

- A bent bone without an obvious fracture. This can occur in young children because the bones are very plastic. The bent bone is referred to as a plastic bowing fracture.
- A dislocation involving the proximal or distal radio-ulnar joint. Characteristically, a displaced fracture of the ulna with an intact radius is accompanied by a dislocated head of the radius – a combination injury known as a Monteggia fracture-dislocation, or a Monteggia lesion. A displaced fracture of the radius with an intact ulna is associated with a dislocation at the distal radio-ulnar joint. This combination injury is known as a Galeazzi fracture-dislocation.

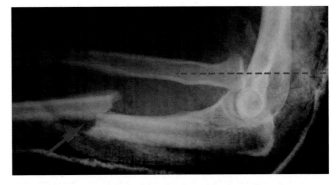

Fracture of the proximal shaft of the ulna (arrow) in plaster. Note the radio-capitellar line is abnormal and indicates an (overlooked) associated dislocation of the head of the radius. This combination injury is known as a Monteggia fracture-dislocation.

Other information

Type of injury and frequency in adults and children

Type of injury	Adults	Children
Fractures		
Supracondylar	• Uncommon	• Common • Most common elbow fracture • Fracture line is usually transverse • Displacement is usually posterior, occasionally anterior • 25% are minimally displaced or undisplaced
Lateral condyle	• Rare	• Common (20% of elbow fractures)
Radial head or neck	• Common • 50% of all fractures at the elbow	• Uncommon
Olecranon	• 20% of elbow injuries • Easy to see	• A normal epiphyseal growth plate can mimic a fracture
Internal epicondyle avulsion	• Not applicable	• Moderate separation – easy to detect • Major separation, with apophysis trapped in joint – easy to overlook. 50% are associated with elbow dislocation
Dislocations		
Elbow	• Common • Invariably – posterior • Often posterolateral	• Uncommon
Head of radius	• Isolated – does occur • Commonly a Monteggia fracture-dislocation injury • Invariably anterior	• Isolated – does occur • Part of a Monteggia fracture-dislocation injury • Invariably anterior
Other		
Pulled elbow	• Rare • May occur in wrestlers	• Common • Age 2-6 years • Annular ligament is stretched and radial head subluxes slightly • Clinical history and examination usually make the diagnosis obvious • Radiography unnecessary as radiographs look normal
Capitellum fracture or dislocation	• Very rare	• Very rare

Particular problems in children

Potential traps	Helpful hints
• Ossifying secondary centres can cause confusion, particularly when a centre shows multicentric ossification • An incompletely fused growth plate can mimic a fracture • A fracture involving the lateral condyle can be dismissed erroneously as the normal apophyseal growth plate • A pulled off medial epicondyle may be trapped in the joint. It can be mistaken for the normal trochlea ossification centre. This lesion is rare but is a recognised complication of a dislocated elbow – even one that has reduced spontaneously	• Doubt or confusion can usually be resolved with the help of a comparison radiograph of the opposite uninjured elbow • Suspect this injury if there is slight widening of the medial joint space on the anteroposterior projection • Remember CRITOE ... and the ossified trochlea never appears before the ossified internal epicondyle

Lines are important, especially in children
Always check the following:

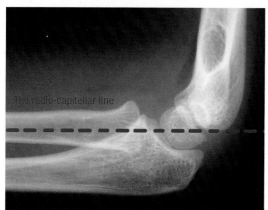

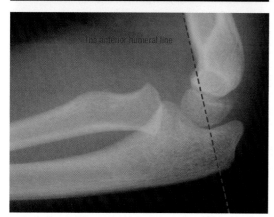

Further reading

Chessare JW, Rogers LF, White H. Injuries of the medial epicondylar ossification center of the humerus. *Am J Roentgenol* 1977;**129**:49-55

Donnelly LF, Klostermeier TT, Klosterman LA. Traumatic elbow effusions in pediatric patients: are occult fractures the rule? *Am J Roentgenol* 1998;**171**:243-5

El-Khoury GY, Daniel WW, Kathol MH. Acute and chronic alvulsive injuries. *Radiol Clin North Am* 1997;**35**:747-66

Fowles JV, Simane N, Kassab MT. Elbow dislocation with avulsion of the medial humeral epicondyle *J Bone Joint Surgery* 1990;**72**:102-4

Gore RM, Rogers LF, Bowerman J, Suker J, Compere CL. Osseous manifestations of elbow stress associated with sports activities. *Am J Roentgenol* 1980;**134**:971-7

Greenspan A, Norman A. The radial head – capitellum view. Useful technique in elbow trauma. *Am J Roentgenol* 1982;**138**:1186-8

Griffith JF, Roebuck DJ, Cheng JC, Chan YL, Rainer TH, Ng BK. Acute elbow trauma in children: spectrum of injury revealed by MR imaging not apparent on radiographs. *Am J Roentgenol* 2001;**176**:53-60

Keats TE. *Atlas of normal roentgen variants that may stimulate disease.* St Louis, CV Mosby, 2001

Miles KA, Finlay DBL. Disruption of the radiocapitellar line in the normal elbow. *Injury* 1989;**20**:365-7

Raby N, Berman L, de Lacey G. *Accident and emergency radiology: a survival guide.* 2nd ed. Philadelphia: Saunders, 2005

Rogers LF. *Radiology of skeletal trauma.* 3rd ed. London: Churchill Livingstone, 2004

Rogers LF, Malave S, White H, Tachdijan MO. Plastic bowing, torus and greenstick supracondylar fracture of the humerus: radiographic clues to obscure fractures of the elbow in children. *Radiology* 1978;**128**:145-50

ABCs systematic assessment – summary

Alignment
• Radio-capitellar line – dislocated radial head
• Anterior humeral line – displaced supracondylar fracture

Bones
• Wrinkles of the cortex – fracture
• Faint depression of the cortex – fracture
• Slight angulation of the cortex – fracture
• Disrupted X sign – supracondylar fracture
• Additional fragment on lateral view. In adults suspect a radio-capitellar fracture or dislocation. In children suspect an avulsed medical epicondyle

Congruity and joints
• Joint spaces not equidistant – dislocated elbow

Soft tissues
• Positive anterior or posterior fat pads – search for a fracture
• No visible fracture but both fat pads displaced. In adults – fracture of the radial head. In children – undisplaced supracondylar fracture

CHAPTER 5

Shoulder

May-ai Seah, David A Elias, Otto Chan

The pectoral girdle suspends the upper limb from the torso, the attachment predominantly being muscular and ligamentous. Soft tissue injury – occult on conventional radiographs – can often be the primary cause of post-traumatic pain and dysfunction. Nevertheless, conventional radiographs are the investigation of choice for the initial evaluation of shoulder trauma, as fracture and dislocation need to be excluded. This chapter reviews the relevant anatomy, radiographic projections, fracture patterns, and some pitfalls that are encountered in the radiographic evaluation of acute shoulder injuries. Other imaging methods, including ultrasonography and magnetic resonance imaging, are predominantly used in the context of more chronic symptoms and suspected soft tissue injuries.

Anatomy

The pectoral girdle includes three bones and three joints. The scapula is a triangular flat bone with a glenoid cavity and coracoid and acromion processes that project laterally. The glenoid cavity is deepened by a fibrocartilaginous ring – the glenoid labrum. This articulates with the humeral head to form the glenohumeral joint. The clavicle and acromioclavicular and sternoclavicular joints complete the pectoral girdle's skeleton.

The humeral head has greater and lesser tuberosities, and the bicipital groove runs between these. The anatomical neck lies superomedial to the tuberosities and the surgical neck below. The appearance and fusion of the secondary ossification centres in children makes the anatomy slightly more confusing, and this can sometimes be confused with a fracture.

The acromioclavicular joint is stabilised by the strong coracoclavicular ligaments and the weaker acromioclavicular ligaments. The glenohumeral joint is stabilised dynamically by the rotator cuff muscles and tendons and statically by the glenohumeral and coracohumeral ligaments. Neurovascular structures, including the axillary vessels and distal branches of the brachial plexus, lie anterior to the glenohumeral joint and may be injured in anterior glenohumeral dislocations or displaced proximal humeral fractures.

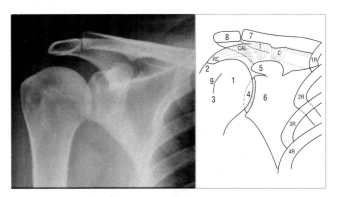

Anteroposterior radiograph (left) and line drawing (right) of shoulder joint. Humerus head (1), greater tuberosity (2), lesser tuberosity (3), glenoid fossa (4), coracoid process (5), neck of scapula (6), clavicle (7), acromion (8), bicipital groove (9), RC=rotator cuff, CAL=coracoacromial ligament, T=trapezoid ligament, C=conoid ligament, R=rib.

Pectoral girdle

Three bones	Three joints
• Scapula	• Glenohumeral
• Humerus	• Acromioclavicular
• Clavicle	• Sternoclavicular

Approximate timings of formation and fusion of secondary ossification centres of the shoulder

Bone	Secondary ossification centre	Time of formation (years)	Time of fusion (years)
Humerus	Head	0-6 months	15-18 (with shaft)
	Greater tuberosity	1	4-6
	Lesser tuberosity	5	7
Scapula	Inferior angle	15	20
	Coracoid	1	15
	Acromion	15	20-25
Clavicle	Medial margin	18	25

ABCs systematic assessment

- Adequacy
- Alignment
- Bone
- Cartilage and joints
- Soft tissues

Adequacy

The anteroposterior radiograph is a routine view for all patients. To profile the glenohumeral joint, this view is normally taken with the patient rotated 15° towards the side of interest. This view should be taken with the arm externally rotated, in which case the greater tuberosity is profiled. As for all skeletal trauma, a minimum of two views is necessary – the second view usually being the axial projection, for which the beam is directed vertically through the shoulder joint with the arm abducted and the cassette placed in the axilla. In the presence of trauma an axial oblique or, alternatively, a "Y" view should be taken because an axial view can be extremely painful.

Various other projections are often used as additional views. Anteroposterior radiographs may be taken with the arm internally rotated, in which case the lesser tuberosity is profiled at the medial humeral head. This is unavoidable in patients with posterior dislocation of the humerus because the arm is fixed in internal rotation and, in this case, the internally rotated appearance of the humeral head is known as the "lightbulb" sign. For assessment of acromioclavicular joint subluxation, weightbearing views that compare the right and left acromioclavicular joints may be needed.

Alignment

Glenohumeral joint

The humeral head should lie in the glenoid fossa, and the distance between the humeral head and the anterior margin of the glenoid should be equal from top to bottom. Loss of this uniform alignment and widening or overlap of the articular surfaces can indicate a dislocation or fracture-dislocation. If the humeral head is also internally rotated and the humeral head looks featureless ("lightbulb sign"), a posterior dislocation should be suspected. Mild inferolateral subluxation of the humeral head may occur with intra-articular fractures because of haemarthrosis or atony of the deltoid muscle.

Acromioclavicular joint

The inferior margins of the lateral end of the clavicle and the acromion should be aligned, although slight malalignment may be seen in up to 20% of healthy people. In such cases, the acromioclavicular joint should not be widened, but if doubt exists, bilateral weightbearing views of the acromioclavicular joints are necessary. Widening of the coracoclavicular distance occurs in patients with acromioclavicular joint dislocation when disruption of the strong coracoclavicular ligaments is present.

Subacromial (acromiohumeral) space

The supraspinatus tendon courses between the inferior margin of the acromion and the superior border of the humeral head. Narrowing of the acromiohumeral distance indicates a massive rotator cuff tear, as loss of this subacromial space can occur only with extensive acute or chronic tears of the supraspinatus and infraspinatus tendons.

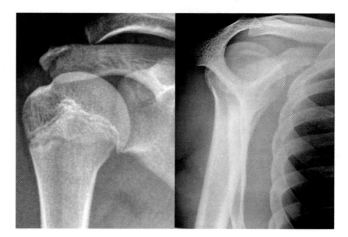

Normal anteroposterior view of a shoulder joint in a child (left) and a normal lateral or "Y" view in an adult (right).

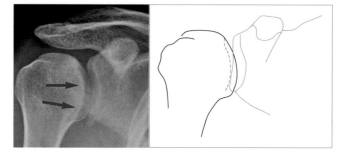

Anteroposterior radiographs of a normal shoulder joint with the arm in external (left) and internal (right) rotation.

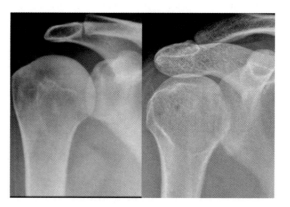

Featureless lightbulb sign with a trough line (arrows). Appearance of the humeral head is consistent with a posterior dislocation.

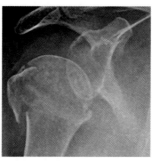

Comminuted fracture of the humeral head with inferior subluxation of the glenohumeral joint caused by a haemarthrosis and/or atony of the deltoid.

Bone

The contour of each bone should be traced systematically. The cortices of the humerus, scapula, clavicle, and ribs should be smooth. Review of the ribs is essential, as fractures of the ribs may be overlooked because of a more obvious fracture of the clavicle or humerus. The internal trabecular pattern of the bones should be examined, and no disruption of the trabecular pattern in the bones should be seen. Subtle fractures should be sought, including impacted fractures of the head or neck of the humerus, Hill-Sachs lesions, or small avulsions from the glenoid rim. These may follow dislocations of the glenhumeral joint.

Interpretation of the axial and Y views follows the same principles as for anteroposterior radiographs. The coracoid process should be identified first. This will identify which side of the film is anterior. The clavicle, lying anteriorly, and the acromion, lying posteriorly, may be identified, and the acromioclavicular joint should be projected over the humeral head in the axial view. The humeral head is identified, and the glenoid and glenohumeral articulation are assessed.

The Y view is helpful to confirm normal alignment of the glenohumeral joint. This view is especially valuable if a posterior dislocation is suspected.

The axial view is useful for assessing glenohumeral alignment, avulsions of the glenoid rim, and Hill-Sachs defects of the humeral head. These subtle fractures may be confirmed with the second view, but further views may be needed.

Cartilage and joints

Check that the joint space is preserved. Apparent narrowing of the joint space is usually the result of technical reasons. True loss of glenohumeral joint space occurs with cartilage loss – most likely because of erosive arthropathies or rarely infection (septic arthritis). Loss of joint space because of primary degenerative disease is uncommon, and an underlying predisposing cause should be excluded through the clinical history. Predisposing causes may include trauma or an underlying erosive arthropathy such as rheumatoid arthritis or haemophilia.

Soft tissues

Acromioclavicular joint disruption usually is associated with adjacent soft tissue swelling. Intra-articular fractures of the glenohumeral joint may occasionally produce a lipohaemarthrosis (fat-fluid level) on an erect anteroposterior radiograph, because of marrow fat leaking into the joint.

Calcification may be seen within the subacromial space in patients with calcific tendonitis of the rotator cuff. Occasionally, a pneumothorax or lung tumour may be identified within the lung in anteroposterior radiographs of the shoulder, so always check the lungs.

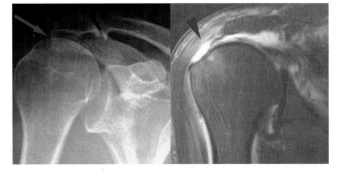

Loss of the subacromial space in anteroposterior radiograph (arrow in left radiograph) and coronal magnetic resonance imaging scan (right) of a chronic supraspinatus tendon rupture (arrowhead).

Normal measurements in anteroposterior radiographs of the shoulder

Feature	Measurement (mm)
Acromioclavicular joint space	≤7; ≤2 for difference between right and left sides
Coracoclavicular separation	≤13
Subacromial space	≥7

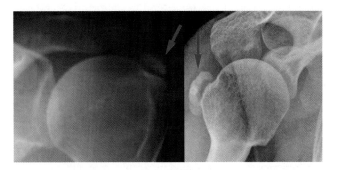

Rotator cuff calcification in the anteroposterior view (arrow in left radiograph) and the axial oblique view (arrow in right radiograph).

Frequency of dislocations about pectoral girdle

Dislocation	Frequency (%)
Glenohumeral (95% anterior; 5% posterior)	85
Acromioclavicular	12
Sternoclavicular	3

Injuries

The pattern of injuries of the shoulder varies with age. Clavicular fractures are a common consequence of birth trauma and are also common in children and young adults. In people aged 15-40 years, glenohumeral and acromioclavicular dislocations are common, whereas humeral head fractures typically occur in older people.

Dislocations
Glenohumeral joint

The glenohumeral joint is the most commonly dislocated joint in the body. Dislocations are classified according to the position of the humeral head with respect to the glenoid, which may be determined from the radiographic series. Associated fractures must be identified.

Anterior dislocations are common and account for over 90% of dislocations of the glenohumeral joint; they may recur in 40% of cases overall and especially in young patients. The diagnosis is usually apparent clinically. The injury typically occurs with abduction and external rotation of the arm and results in a clinically "squared off" appearance of the shoulder and a prominent acromion process. The humeral head may be palpable in the anterior axilla. Radiographically, the humeral head typically lies anterior, medial, and inferior with respect to the glenoid. The dislocation is usually obvious on the anteroposterior view alone, but a second view is always taken to exclude a fracture. A compression fracture of the posterolateral aspect of the humeral head, known as a Hill-Sachs defect, occurs because of impaction against the anterior glenoid and is reported in more than 50% of cases. It is seen as a bony defect on the anteroposterior view taken with internal rotation or in the axial or axial oblique views. About 15% of cases may be associated with fractures of the greater tuberosity and around 8% with fractures of the anteroinferior bony glenoid – Bankart's defect.

Posterior dislocations of the glenohumeral joint are rare (<10% of dislocations of the joint). As clinical and radiographic signs are subtle, more than half of cases may be missed initially, with resulting chronic pain and immobility. Dislocation occurs with a posterior force on the humeral head in internal rotation. Seizures are the most common cause, and, in such cases, dislocation may be bilateral. Associated fractures are common. Rare forms of glenohumeral dislocation include superior dislocation, inferior dislocation (luxatio erecta), and intrathoracic dislocation.

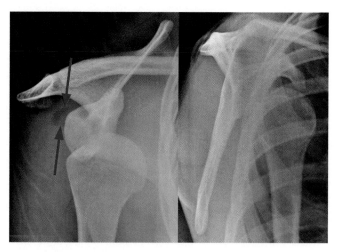

Anterior dislocation of glenohumeral joint in the anteroposterior view (left) and Y view (right). Note the lipohaemarthrosis (arrows) on the anteroposterior view that implies there must be an intra-articular fracture also (not visible).

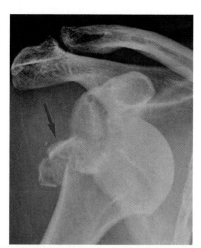

Anterior dislocation on anteroposterior view with a comminuted fracture (arrow) of the greater tuberosity.

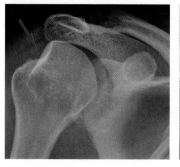

Hill-Sach's defect (arrow) on the anteroposteriori view taken with the arm in internal rotation in a patient who had a previous anterior dislocation (now reduced).

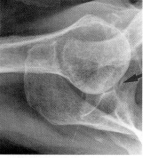

Bony Bankart's defect (arrow) of the anterior glenoid with anterior dislocation of the humeral head on an axial view.

Signs of posterior glenohumeral dislocation

- Lightbulb sign – humeral head fixed in severe internal rotation
- Rim sign – joint space between medial border of the humeral head and anterior glenoid rim >6 mm
- Incongruity of the humeral head and the glenoid fossa
- Trough line – sclerotic line paralleling the medial cortex of the humeral head because of an impaction fracture of the antero-medial head
- Fracture of the lesser tuberosity

Acromioclavicular joint

Injuries of the acromioclavicular joint are of variable severity, and this is reflected in the Rockwood classification. Type I injuries are normal radiographically, whereas type II injuries may be visible only in stress views.

Sternoclavicular joint

Sternoclavicular dislocation is uncommon and is difficult to diagnose radiographically because of overlapping structures. On an anteroposterior radiograph of the chest, the medial clavicles lie at different levels. Dislocation is usually anterosuperior, but the rarer posterosuperior dislocation is important because of potential injury to mediastinal structures and pneumothorax.

Fractures

Clavicle

Clavicular fractures are common, usually after falls onto the shoulder or outstretched hand. About 80% occur in the middle third, with over-riding of the fracture and inferior displacement of the distal fragment. Occasionally, subclavian neurovascular injuries occur. Fractures of the lateral aspect are less common and are often undisplaced because of stabilisation from the coracoclavicular ligaments.

Clavicular fractures may occur during birth – especially with breech presentations. Callus formation is seen at 8-9 days. Ageing the fracture may help distinguish injuries caused during birth from non-accidental injuries.

Scapula

Fractures of the body of the scapula usually require severe trauma and have a significant association with injuries of the head, thorax, and spine. Fractures of the acromion may occur because of a direct blow. Coracoid fractures occasionally occur after glenohumeral dislocation.

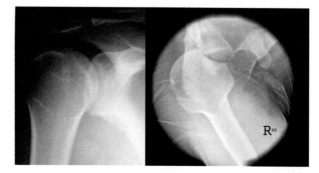

Posterior dislocation in anteroposterior view (lightbulb sign) (left) and an axial view (right).

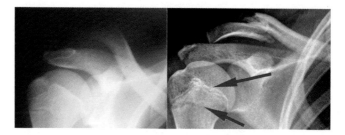

Acromioclavicular joint dislocation (left) and clavicle fracture (right) in a child. Note the proximal humeral growth plate that undulates and so is seen at two levels (arrows). This should not be confused with a fracture.

Rockwood classification of acromioclavicular joint injury

Type	Injury	Radiographic appearance
I	Minor injury to acromioclavicular ligament	Normal
II	Acromioclavicular ligaments disrupted; coracoclavicular ligaments intact	Widened acromioclavicular joint; normal coracoclavicular distance
III	Acromioclavicular and coracoclavicular ligaments disrupted	Widened acromioclavicular joint and coracoclavicular distance
IV	Posterior dislocation with buttonholing of lateral clavicle through trapezius	Acromioclavicular joint widening; essentially a clinical diagnosis
V	As III, but with severe upward displacement of clavicle	Severe upward displacement of clavicle
VI	Inferior displacement of clavicle	Clavicle lies inferior to coracoid

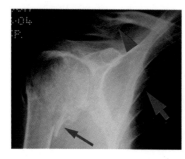

Fracture at neck of humerus. Note old healed clavicle (arrow) and rib fractures (arrowhead) in an alcoholic.

Proximal humerus

Proximal humeral fractures show two peaks of incidence:

- In adolescents because of epiphyseal separation
- In people aged >45 years because of osteoporosis.

In adults, fractures most commonly involve the surgical neck, and comminution may occur, with involvement of the tuberosities or the anatomical neck. Acute complications include neurovascular injury, while delayed complications include adhesive capsulitis and, with fractures of the anatomical neck, avascular necrosis of the humeral head. Humeral shaft fractures are common and may be associated with radial nerve injury in up to 17% of cases.

ABCs systematic assessment

Alignment

- Check glenohumeral joint
  Inferomedial displacement
  indicates anterior dislocation
  Lightbulb and trough line indicates posterior dislocation
  Inferolateral subluxation
  indicates haemarthrosis
- Check acromioclavicular joint
  for
  Widening of acromioclavicular
  joint
  Widening of corococlavicular
  distance
- Check acromiohumeral
  distance
  <7mm indicates massive rotator cuff tear

Bone

- Check for fractures
  A trough line indicates posterior dislocation
  In an anteriror dislocation of
  the glenohumeral joint take
  a second view to exclude a
  fracture.
  These fractures may include
  a posterolateral defect in
  humeral head (Hill-Sach's
  defect) or an anteroinferior
  glenoid fracture (Bankart's
  defect)

Cartilage and joints

- Check for loss of joint space
- Check for erosive arthropathy or degerative changes,
  especially if there is a history
  of rheumatoid arthritis or
  haemophilia

Soft tissues

- Rotator cuff calcification
  indicates calcific tendonitis
- Lipohaemarthrosis (fat-fluid
  level) indicates intra-articular
  fracture
- Exclude lung pathology – for
  example, pneumothorax or
  haemothorax

Neer classification of proximal humeral fractures

- Fractures may extend through the surgical neck, greater or lesser tuberosities, or anatomical neck
- Displacement across a fracture = separation >1 cm or angulation >45°

Type	Description	Frequency (%)
One part	No substantial displacement across fracture lines; considered stable	80
Two part	Displacement across one fracture	10
Three part	Some displacement across two fractures	3
Four part	Serious displacement across three fractures; severe comminution; avascular necrosis likely	4

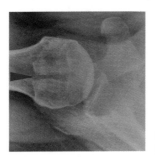

Os acromiale – normal accessory ossicle (arrowhead).

Normal variants not to be confused with pathology

- Bicipital groove: appears as a sclerotic line. Do not confuse it with fracture
- In children, the anterior and posterior aspects of the proximal humeral growth plate are at different levels in the anteroposterior view. Do not confuse it with fracture
- Decreased density of the superolateral humeral head is a normal finding not a bone cyst
- Rhomboid fossa: a normal concavity at the inferomedial clavicle that may be asymmetric, and can look like an aggressive lesion
- Os acromiale: unfused accessory ossicle (present in 10% of people). Do not confuse with a fracture of the acromion

KEY POINTS

- Anterior dislocation is easy to diagnose
- Posterior dislocation is a difficult diagnosis to make. Always confirm with a second view (Y view)
- If the patient has localised pain, and an injury to the acromio-clavicular joint is suspected, then get weight bearing views
- Always check the scapula, ribs, and the underlying lung.

CHAPTER 6

Pelvis and Hip

James A S Young, Jeremy W R Young, Otto Chan

Pelvic fractures that result from major trauma are life threatening injuries, and they are often associated with other injuries. The biomechanics of such injuries mean that the hip may have touched the opposite shoulder – that is, the patient may also have a head, spine, chest, abdominal or limb injury. Remember that pelvic radiographs represent the final position of rest and that only bony injuries are seen.

A fracture is a soft tissue injury in which the bone happens to have been injured – this applies particularly to fractures of the pelvis, which is a major site for occult bleeding after major trauma. Apart from possible major intra-abdominal and vascular injuries, the internal pelvic organs are often injured – particularly the bladder, urethra, and rectum and, in women, the vagina, cervix, and uterus.

Hip fractures, on the other hand, usually occur in elderly patients and may represent a relatively minor injury. A hip fracture in a young patient, however, usually indicates that the patient has sustained major trauma.

Anatomy

Bony anatomy

Pelvis

Essentially, the pelvis is composed of a bony ring that consists of three bones – the sacrum and two innominate bones held together by several ligaments. The most important are the sacroiliac ligaments, which are the strongest ligaments in the body and provide stability to the pelvic ring.

The three bones of the pelvis can be separated only when the ligaments are torn. When this happens, the nerves and vessels running close to them may also be damaged. In addition, all the other soft tissues and organs within the abdomen and pelvis may be injured. Bleeding is usually venous and extraperitoneal, but it can be arterial and can be life threatening. If the bones fracture but the ligaments remain intact, a tamponade effect can be achieved and the degree of haemorrhage can be limited.

Hip

In adults the strong hip joint capsule and the surrounding large muscle bulk prevent dislocation except in cases of severe trauma. More commonly, the hip is fractured, and this may be associated with avascular necrosis of the femoral head, particularly complicating intracapsular fractures, and epiphyseal injuries. The trochanteric

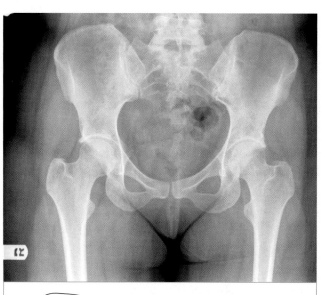

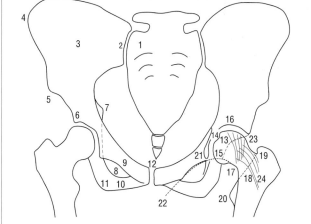

Normal anteroposterior view of pelvis and hip in an adult. The pelvis is labelled on the left side of the figure: sacrum (1), sacroiliac joint (2), ilium (3), iliac crest (4), anterior superior iliac spine (5), anterior inferior iliac spine (6), ischial spine (7), obdurator foramen (8), superior pubic ramus (9), inferior pubic ramus (10), ischial tuberosity (11), pubic symphysis (12). The hip is labelled on the right side of the figure: femoral head (13), fovea capitis (14), acetabular margin (15), acetabulum (16), neck of femur (17), intertrochanteric line (18), greater trochanter (19), lesser trochanter (20), Kohler's tear drop (21), Shenton's line (22), compressive trabeculae (23), tensile trabeculae (24).

apophyses are the insertion points for the gluteus medius (greater trochanter) and iliopsoas (lesser trochanter) muscles and are prone to avulsion in athletic adolescents. In malignant disease, the proximal femur, particularly the subtrochanteric region, is a common site for metastases and pathological fracture.

In children the proximal capital femoral epiphysis is present from the age of three months until 18-20 years, with double epiphyseal ossification centres being common. Although asymmetry, irregular contour, and notching of the epiphyses can be normal variants in young children, a smaller epiphysis or any asymmetry in children with symptoms in the hips may indicate injury. Flattening or an abnormal contour or widening of the epiphysis is abnormal. The metaphysis has a rich blood supply and is a common site for osteomyelitis and thus septic arthritis.

ABCs systematic assessment

- **A**dequacy
- **A**lignment
- **B**one
- **C**artilage and joints
- **S**oft tissues

Pelvis

Adequacy

In most cases, a correct diagnosis can be made only from an anteroposterior radiograph of the pelvis. It gives a good overall assessment and allows for diagnosis of most overtly destructive or traumatic processes. In cases of trauma, inlet and outlet views are useful, especially if there are displaced fractures. Oblique (Judet) views are preferred in cases of acetabular injury.

If computed tomography is available immediately, it is generally the preferred diagnostic tool. Computed tomography is particularly useful in cases of acetabular injury, where it is superior to plain radiography. It can define the pattern of injury, especially with multiplanar imaging, and it can also detect small intra-articular bone fragments.

If computed tomography is not available, inlet and outlet views should be requested if clinical or radiologic evidence suggests a pelvic fracture. An inlet view looks down the lumen of the true pelvis and is better than the anteroposterior view for showing the orientation of fractures of the pubic rami. Outlet views are used to detect the degree of vertical displacement of fracture fragments.

When examining the radiographs, check the adequacy and quality of the film. Ensure that the whole of the pelvis can be seen, including the iliac crests, both hips, and the greater and lesser trochanters. This ideal is not always possible in patients with multiple trauma. The adequacy of the radiographic penetration should be assessed because correct exposure of the pelvis in elderly patients (who often have large bellies and thin upper thighs) can be difficult. Usually, the pelvis is exposed properly, but the hips and, particularly the greater trochanters, are extremely dark, and a bright light needs to be used or a separate radiograph taken. Pelvic rotation is determined by lining up the symphysis pubis with the midline of the sacrum and checking the symmetry of the obdurator foramen. Often, part of the

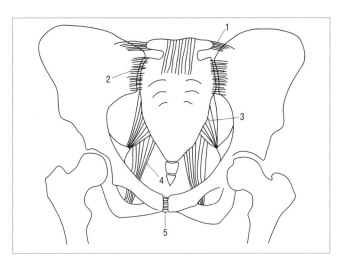

Major supporting ligaments of pelvis: (1) posterior sacroiliac ligament; (2) right anterior sacroiliac ligament; (3) left sacrospinous ligament; (4) right sacrotuberous ligament; (5) pubic symphysis.

Radiographic projections of pelvis and hip

Pelvis	Hip
Standard	*Standard*
• Anteroposterior view of hips	• Anteroposterior view of both hips
	• Lateral
Additional	*Additional*
• Judet view	• Frog leg lateral view
• Inlet view	
• Outlet view	

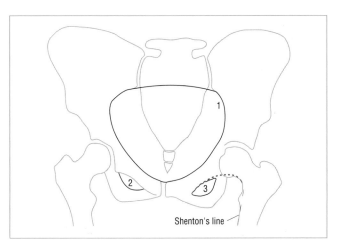

Normal pelvis with three circles and Shenton's line.

iliac crest is missing or the film is penetrated poorly so that fractures cannot be seen. A rotated film causes asymmetry of the bony circles and sacroiliac joints.

Alignment and bones

The pelvic bones are made up of three circles. One circle is created by the pelvic rim and the other two by the obturator foramina. A line drawn around the pelvic brim should be followed. Normally this has a smooth edge that is not disrupted by the sacroiliac joint or pubic symphysis unless the patient is very old. If a fracture is detected, always check for a second disruption in the circle because there is nearly always another fracture or diastasis. (Imagine a polo mint – it is difficult to break it in one place only). As the pelvis is not completely rigid, a second disruption in the circle may take the form of a minimal diastasis, which may be extremely subtle and can be difficult to see on frontal radiographic views.

Avulsion fractures as a result of ligamentous strain have the same effect as ruptures of the corresponding ligaments. Although quite rare, they are important to detect in plain radiographs. For example, avulsion of the lateral border of the sacrum or ischial spine indicates an anteroposterior compression force sufficient to compromise the sacroiliac ligament and sacrotuberous-sacrospinous complex.

The inner margins of both obturator foramina should then be inspected in the same way as the pelvic brim. Complete the examination of the foramina by tracing along the inferior border of the pubic ramus and then along the medial aspect of the neck of the femur. This is Shenton's line. Disruption of this normally smooth line indicates that the femoral neck is broken. Remember, however, that non-displaced femoral neck fractures may be difficult to see.

The cortical margins of the pelvic bones should be examined for evidence of fractures. These are usually obvious and present as areas of increased density, lucency, or alteration of internal trabecular pattern.

Start the examination by gaining an overview of the entire pelvis, which will define asymmetry, displacement, and most fractures. A more detailed secondary search is then conducted, starting at the pubic symphysis and progressing to the right and left iliac wings, including the acetabula. The search is completed at the sacrum, with particular interest in the intrasacral segment anastomoses and neural foramina. Interruption of these lines is strong evidence of a fracture. Several lines are useful in examination of the acetabulum. These are the iliopectineal line (outline the posterior column), the ilioischial line (outlines the anterior column), and the teardrop line (outlines the medial wall of the acetabulum).

Epiphyseal lines may be misinterpreted as fractures. Remember that the Y shaped (triradiate) cartilage that separates the pubis, ischium, and ilium in the acetabular floor does not fuse until puberty. Accessory ossification centres (in particular, the centre in the posterior acetabulum) may also be mistaken for fractures. Apophyses, however, are usually bilateral, have a sclerotic margin, and are not associated with overlying soft tissue signs.

Fractures in the acetabulum can be detected by tracing over the cortical margins and the various lines described above. Posterior and anterior acetabular rim fractures can be missed easily because they are covered by the femoral head. Look for isolated bone fragments lying behind the femoral head.

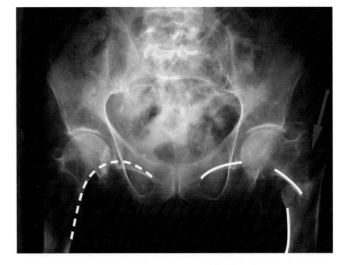

Fracture at neck of femur with displaced Shenton's line.

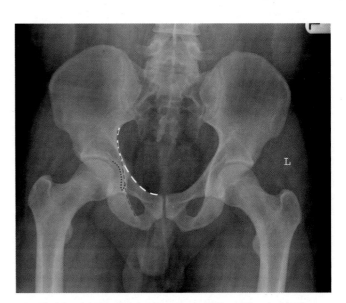

Normal adult pelvis showing the three acetabular lines. When looking for acetabular fractures the iliopectoneal (arcuate) line (shown as a dashed white line), ilioischial line (shown as a red dashed line), and the teardrop line (shown by a blue dotted line) aid diagnosis.

Cartilage and joints

Pubic symphysis can be detected by checking for widening or overlapping of bone. Such an injury may be associated with disruption elsewhere in the pelvic brim: this is dependent on the force vector that caused the injury.

Check the right and left sides of the sacroiliac joints for widening, defects in the cortical surface, overlapping of bone, and lack of congruity of the joint margin. This may be seen more easily on an inlet view. Computed tomography, however, is the method of choice for definitive evaluation of these joints.

Soft tissues

Although a check of the soft tissues is important, only gross abnormality is seen on plain radiographs. Check for soft tissue shadowing inside and outside the pelvis because haematoma and tissue oedema can produce swellings that are visible in anteroposterior radiographs. Normally, the obturator internus muscle is seen on both sides of the pelvis as a dark grey line that is the result of the muscle or fat plane. Loss or displacement of this line may indicate a fracture. The bladder outline should also be visible, and displacement or asymmetry of the perivesical fat plane often indicates a fracture.

Patterns of injury to the pelvis

Four patterns of force lead to pelvic damage:

• Lateral compression: force vector is delivered from the side. It is the most common form of fracture and usually occurs as a result of broadside traffic accidents or a fall onto the side. It produces horizontal fractures or "buckle" fractures of the pubic rami, which are often associated with a crush fracture of the sacrum and a momentary medial displacement of the hemipelvis. The extent of this movement depends on the amount of force and point of impact. A lateral compression force can also impinge on the upper femur, resulting in central dislocation of the hip or a crush fracture of the femoral neck.

• Anteroposterior compression: force comes from the front (or from behind). It is caused by a frontal force that causes vertical fractures of the pubic rami or tends to cause one or both sides of the pelvis to open up like a book, with the spine of the "book" running down the sacrum. A combination of these injuries may also occur. Mild diastasis of the symphysis pubis can occur with disruption of the ligaments of the synphysis alone, but for the pubic bones to separate by more than 2.5 cm, the ligamentous groups of at least the anterior sacroiliac joints have to be torn. In addition, disruption of the more inferior sacrospinous or sacrotuberous ligaments will cause further instability, and, if the posterior sacroiliac ligaments are disrupted, complete separation of the iliac wing can occur. Severe anteroposterior compression fractures will therefore cause marked pelvic instability. An anteroposterior force can also push the flexed femur backward so that the femoral head may dislocate or fracture of the posterior acetabular rim or wall may occur.

• Vertical shear: force is delivered in the vertical plane, as in a fall from a height. Vertical shear forces the hemipelvis upwards and results in vertical fractures of the iliac wing and pubic rami or disruption of the sacroiliac ligaments on the affected side as well as the ligaments of the pubic symphysis, or both, with superior displace-

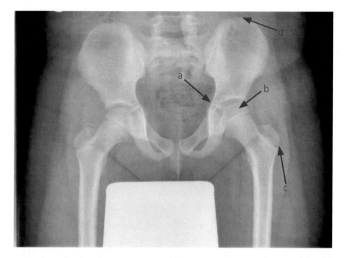

Normal paediatric pelvis in a 10 year old boy. Note the normal epiphyseal growth lines of the triradiate cartilage of the acetabulum (a), the superior femoral epiphysis (b), and the trochanteric apophysis of the greater trochanter (c). The iliac apophysis (d) does not appear until puberty, and it is the last growth plate in the body to fuse, usually at about 20 years.

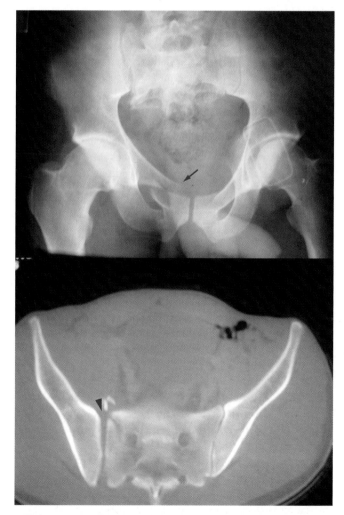

Lateral compression fracture – In the top radiograph horizontal fracture lines are seen in the pubic rami (arrow) on the right with diastasis of the right sacro-iliac joint with a subtle fracture of the right sacrum (arrowhead). The axial computed tomogram (bottom) confirms the diatasis of the right sacro-iliac joint with a crush fracture of the sacrum (arrowhead).

ment of the fractured hemipelvic fragment. This is associated with severe pelvic instability and vascular or other soft tissue damage.
- Complex pattern: in some cases, the pelvis is subjected to a combination of forces mentioned above. A combination of injuries results in a complex radiologic pattern. Nevertheless, radiographs can usually still be interpreted using the principles mentioned.
- Pelvic damage can also be caused by a combination of two or more of the above.

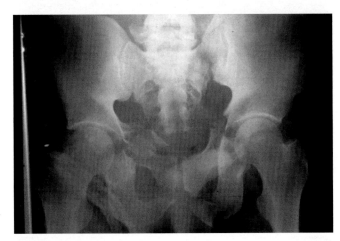

A serious vertical shear injury.

Hip

Adequacy

When a hip injury is suspected, request an anteroposterior view of both hips and a lateral view of the affected hip. The anteroposterior view of the hips is similar to the anteroposterior view of the pelvis, except that it is centred lower. This means that the top of the iliac crest is not usually included, but the upper thirds of the femurs are. A view of the whole lower pelvis is taken when a hip injury is suspected on one side because the symptoms may be caused by a pubic ring injury on the same or opposite side.

Apart from the standard views of the pelvis and hips, the frog leg lateral film is useful in children. It shows the femoral head and neck in a position between the anteroposterior and the standard lateral projection. Anteroposterior and lateral views of the femoral shaft and knee are indicated when the patient has a history of severe trauma or when clinical findings suggest more than one fracture site.

Anteroposterior view of hip

Check bone margins and density – Trace around the margin of the proximal femur, starting at the inferior aspect of the medial femoral cortex and checking for any disruption of the cortical line, particularly around the neck or trochanters. In patients who can bear weight, carefully examine the trabecular lines and cortical margins of the femoral neck in a coned anteroposterior film to detect undisplaced fractures. Undisplaced femoral neck fractures will have a discontinuity in the trabecular lines, with an associated linear increase in density when impacted. Check the cortical lines of the acetabular joint surface and posterior and anterior rim. Both hips should be symmetrical.

Cartilage and joints – In children, widening of the joint space between the teardrop and the cortex of the femoral head may be seen in joint effusions. A difference of more than 2 mm between the two

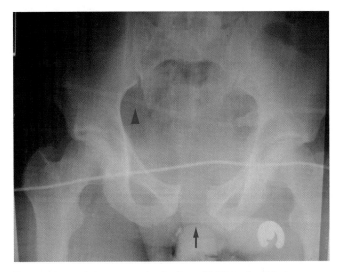

Severe anteroposterior compression fracture with bilateral acetabular fractures and with diastasis of the symphysis pubis and right sacro-iliac joint.

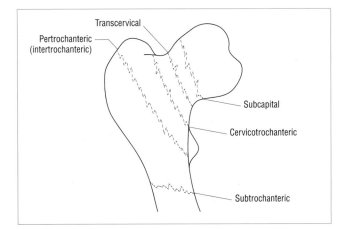

Sites of fracture of the femoral neck.

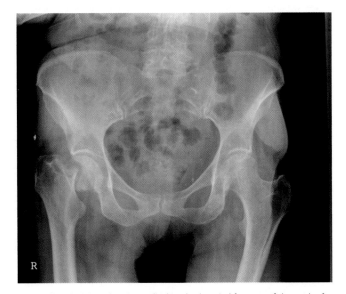

Anteroposterior view showing a displaced subcapital fracture of the neck of the femur.

sides is important clinically. Check that the physis (growth plate) is not widened or compressed (Salter-Harris types I and V fractures).

Check soft tissues – Because of the large muscle mass around the hip, soft tissue injuries are not visible in plain radiographs. Air or a metallic foreign body will be seen after a penetrating injury. If air is seen to outline the femoral head or acetabulum, the joint capsule has been breached.

Lateral projection of hip

Check adequacy and quality of radiograph – Cross table lateral film should include acetabulum, ischial spine and tuberosity, and proximal femur. The trochanters overlap. In the frog leg lateral film, the greater trochanter should project over the neck of the femur. The lateral view may be difficult to evaluate and is of limited value. Computed tomography is often the preferred choice if the clinical diagnosis is difficult and initial imaging is equivocal.

Anteroposterior and lateral views of the femoral shaft and knee are indicated in patients with a history of severe trauma or when clinical findings suggest more than one site of fracture. Gonad protection should always be used in children and adults of reproductive age, as long as it will not obscure a fracture.

Check alignment of bones – Femoral neck lies anteverted about 30° to the femoral shaft. Check that the entire metaphysis is covered by the epiphysis in children and adolescents. In a slipped upper femoral epiphysis, the centre of the femoral metaphysis lies anterior to its normal position over the central epiphysis. In patients with dislocated hips, the cross table lateral film will define whether dislocation is anterior or posterior.

Check bone margins and density – Trace around the margins of the femur and then the acetabulum and ischium. If a dislocation is present, look for acetabular fragments. These are usually displaced in the same direction as the femoral head.

Check soft tissues – Accessory ossification centres, recognised by their corticated margins, are common around the acetabular margins and may simulate fractures when partially fused in adolescence. They may persist into adult life. Acetabular roof notches and roof asymmetry are recognised normal variants. Symmetrical protrusion of the acetabular roofs medially is common in children aged 4-12 years.

Hypertrophic changes of the femoral head or inferior aspect of the neck may simulate fractures. Skin folds superimposed over the intertrochanteric region extend past the outer cortical margins, and this differentiates them from fractures. In early childhood, the trabecula of the femoral neck may produce a striated pattern or unusual lucencies that simulate osteoporosis. If the plain film shows no abnormality in children who present with an irritable hip, other imaging is indicated, and orthopaedic referral is mandatory.

Femoral neck fractures

Femoral neck fractures are most often seen after a fall in older women with osteopenia, although they also are seen in patients who have major pelvic trauma. Fractures occur at four sites. Fractures may be intracapsular or extracapsular, and they are usually visible in the anteroposterior film as a lucent line. The fracture line may be sclerotic, however, particularly if some impaction of the trabecu-

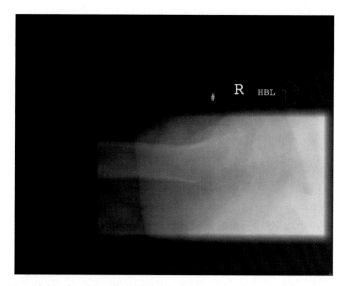

Lateral view showing a displaced subcapital fracture of the neck of the femur.

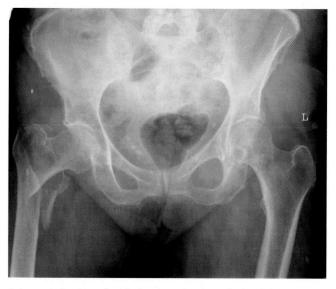

Anteroposterior view of pelvis showing a showing a displaced, three part, intertrochanteric fracture of the femur.

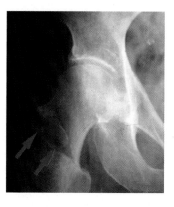

Lucent fracture at the neck of femur.

lae has occurred. Pertrochanteric (intertrochanteric) fractures are often comminuted, with displacement of the lesser trochanter being present.

The subcapital fractures are also classified by the severity extent of the injury. This is important because the classification will decide the management of the fracture.

Garden's classification of subcapital fractures

- Grade I – incomplete fracture
- Grade II – complete fracture but no displacement
- Grade III – some separation of fracture
- Grade IV – complete separation of fracture

In children, considerable violence is needed to fracture the neck of the femur. In transepiphyseal fractures, the capital epiphysis is separated from the metaphysis and dislocated out of the acetabulum; this often results in avascular necrosis.

Delbet classification of femoral neck fractures in children

- Type 1 – transepiphyseal (avascular necrosis usually follows)
- Type 2 – transcervical (avascular necrosis common if displaced)
- Type 3 – cervicotrochanteric
- Type 4 – pertrochanteric

Acetabular fractures

Acetabular fractures may occur because of injury to the pelvic ring or they may occur separately. Fractures of the posterior rim are usually caused by posterior dislocation of the femur and are therefore often seen in anteroposterior compression fractures of the pelvis. Posterior wall fractures are also common in anteroposterior compression injuries. Less common anterior pillar fractures are seen in anteroposterior compression fractures of the pelvis, usually as a result of direct trauma to the anterior pelvis. Fractures of the quadrilateral plate, however, generally occur after lateral compression fractures and are often part of a more complex pattern of acetabular injury that usually involves the posterior pillar or anterior pillar, or both. Acetabular fractures may be complicated by sciatic nerve palsy and by severe intrapelvic haemorrhage.

Acetabular fractures

In general, acetabular fractures involve one or more of four regions:
- Posterior rim
- Posterior pillar
- Anterior pillar
- Medial wall (quadrilateral plate)

Dislocation

The femoral head can be dislocated anteriorly, posteriorly, or centrally. Central dislocation occurs when the femoral head impacts through the acetabulum because of a sideways fall, a blow to the greater trochanter, or a fall from a height onto the feet. Falling onto the feet is often associated with a vertical fracture of the anterior or

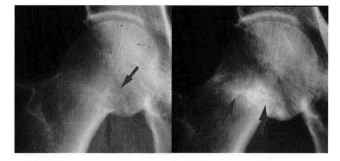

Subtle sclerotic fracture of the right neck of femur (arrow) at presentation (left), and two weeks later (right).

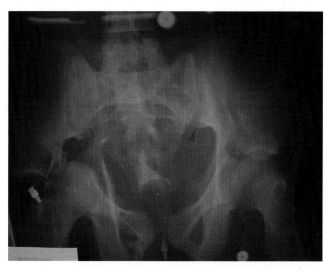

Severe anteroposterior compression fracture with bilateral acetabular fractures and marked displacement of the fragments on the right. Diastasis of the left sacroiliac joint and separation of the pubic symphysis are seen.

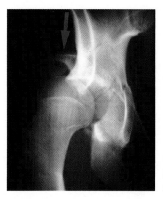

Dislocated femoral head with associated acetabular fracture.

posterior pelvic columns. Posterior dislocation may result from a blow to the lumbar spine – for example, from falling masonry – with the hip flexed. In patients who have hit a car's dashboard, dislocation of the hip is often associated with fracture of the femoral shaft or patella.

Complications of hip dislocation

- Slipped femoral epiphysis (unfused skeleton)
- Sciatic nerve palsy
- Femoral nerve or artery compression (anterior dislocation)
- Failed reduction and recurrent dislocation
- Avascular necrosis of the femoral head
- Osteoarthritis
- Myositis ossificans
- In severe trauma, fractures of the patella and femoral shaft, neck, or head often occur in combination with central dislocation of the hip

Congenital dislocation of the hip

Successful treatment depends on correct and early recognition of this condition. Ultrasonography is the preferred method of diagnosis; however, diagnosis can be made from plain radiographs. At birth, the femoral epiphysis is not ossified, but the acetabular roof is often abnormal, with notching laterally and an increased acetabular angle. Once the epiphysis is ossified, the disorder becomes obvious from radiography.

Idiopathic coxa vara

Idiopathic coxa vara is part of a spectrum of conditions known as proximal femoral focal deficiency of which two types exist: congenital and infantile. Lesions are usually bilateral and present with coxa vara with epiphysis that is low lying and looks "woolly", and there is epiphyseal or metaphyseal lucency.

Slipped capital femoral epiphysis (adolescent coxa vara)

In this condition, the femoral neck moves proximally and externally rotates on the unfused epiphysis. In 20% of cases the condition is bilateral, and it occurs in overweight, hypogonadal, or tall but thin adolescents. Pain, sometimes referred to the knee, or limp is a common presenting symptom. Both hips should be evaluated. Early slip is best assessed in the frog leg lateral film.

KEY POINTS

- Pelvic fractures caused by major trauma are life threatening
- In patients with pelvic fractures, suspect vascular, abdominal, and pelvic organ injuries (especially of the bladder, urethra, and rectum)
- If a pelvic ring fracture is found, always look for a second fracture
- Hip fractures in older patients are common and may be difficult to detect. Always use a bright light

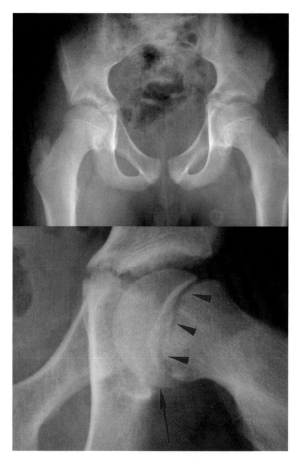

Slipped capital femoral epiphysis – Anteroposterior view (top) appears normal. Frog leg lateral view (bottom) shows the slipped capital femoral epiphysis (arrow) and widening of the epiphyseal growth plate (arrowheads).

ABCs systematic assessment

Adequacy
- Ensure that all the pelvis and hips are visible
- Use a bright light to look carefully at the hips and iliac crest
- Use one view for the pelvis and two views for the hips

Alignment
- Check three rings – main pelvic brim and two obturator foramina
- Check hip joints
- Check Shenton's line

Bone
- Check each of the following systematically:
  Pelvis, pubis, and sacrum
  Iliac crest and lumbar vertebrae
  Acetabulum, femoral head, and femur
  Trabecular lines
- Note: If you see one pelvic ring fracture, there is probably another

Cartilage and joints
- Check the pubic symphysis
- Check the sacroiliac joints
- Check the hip joints and acetabulum

Soft tissues
- Check the obturator internus fat planes inside the pelvis
- Check the perivesical fat plane
- Check the femoral pulses and sciatic nerve

CHAPTER 7

Knee

Rashika Fernando, David A Elias, Otto Chan

Conventional radiographs are the usual initial imaging investigation in patients who present with knee trauma. Knee stability is maintained by ligamentous and musculotendinous structures, so severe injury may be present with little or no abnormality in conventional radiographs. Techniques such as ultrasonography and magnetic resonance imaging are often needed to evaluate such injuries. Ultrasonography enables evaluation of effusions and bursae and assessment of injury to the extensor mechanism as well as to superficial ligaments. Magnetic resonance imaging allows comprehensive assessment of soft tissue and bony injuries. As appropriate expertise and equipment becomes available, ultrasonography and magnetic resonance imaging are used more often in the early evaluation of knee injuries. The use of computed tomography in patients with acute knee trauma, primarily for assessment of the degree of depression of tibial plateau fractures, is well established.

Anatomy

The knee is a hinge-type synovial joint formed by articulation between the femoral condyles and tibial plateau. The two bones are separated by two C shaped fibrocartilaginous structures: the medial and lateral menisci. Along with the hyaline cartilage, which lines the articular surfaces of the femoral condyles and tibial plateau, these create the medial and lateral joint space seen on weightbearing radiographic images of the knee.

The patella is a large sesamoid bone in the knee extensor mechanism. The quadriceps muscles form the quadriceps tendon, which inserts into the superior pole of the patella. The patella tendon extends from the inferior patella pole to insert onto the tibial tuberosity. The posterior surface of the patella has a wide lateral facet and a small medial facet for articulation with the trochlear groove on the anterior surface of the femoral condyles and to form the patellofemoral joint. The fibular head and posterolateral proximal tibia articulate at the proximal tibiofibular joint.

Ottowa decision rule* for radiography in knee injury

Radiographs of the knee are needed only in the presence of more than one of:
- Age >55 years
- Tenderness at fibula head
- Isolated tenderness of patella
- Inability to flex to 90°
- Inability to bear weight for four steps immediately after injury and in emergency department

*The rule is positive in 98-100% of patients with fractures.

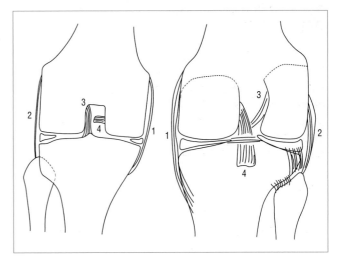

Anatomy of the right knee shown in anterior view (left) and posterior view (right). Medial collateral ligament (1), lateral collateral ligament (2), anterior cruciate ligament (3), posterior cruciate ligament (4).

Secondary ossification centres about the knee

Bone	Secondary ossification centre	At formation	At fusion
		Age (years)	
Femur	Distal femoral epiphysis	Birth–2 months	15-17
Tibia	Proximal tibial epiphysis	Birth–2 months	15-17
	Tibial tuberosity apophysis	8-14	15 (with metaphysis)
Patella	May have multiple centres	3-6	
Fibula	Proximal fibula epiphysis	3-4	15-17

Ligaments and musculotendinous structures provide the knee with stability. The knee is surrounded by multiple bursae. The suprapatellar bursa is continuous with the knee joint and lies between the suprapatellar fat and prefemoral fat above the level of the patella. A Baker's cyst lies in the popliteal fossa and has a neck that insinuates between the tendons of the medial head of gastrocnemius and semimembranosus. The neck may communicate with the joint. The popliteal artery and vein lie in the popliteal fossa and are vulnerable to trauma after certain injuries, such as some supracondylar femoral fractures and knee dislocations. The common peroneal nerve winds around the fibular neck and may be damaged in injuries of the lateral leg.

Supporting ligaments and musculotendinous structures

Structure	Origin	Insertion	Primary function
Anterior cruciate ligament	Posterolateral aspect of roof of intercondylar notch of femur	Anterior intercondylar eminence of tibia	Resists anterior translation and internal rotation of tibia
Posterior cruciate ligament	Anteromedial intercondylar notch of femur	Posterior tibial eminence	Resists posterior displacement and external rotation of tibia
Medial collateral ligament	Medial epicondyle of femur	Medial proximal tibial metaphysis	Resists valgus stress
Lateral collateral ligament	Lateral epicondyle of femur	Fibular head	Resists varus stress
Quadriceps mechanism	Anterior pelvis and proximal femur	Tibial tuberosity	Knee extension and patellar stabilisation

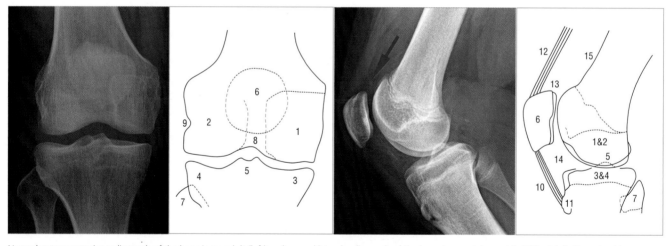

Normal anteroposterior radiograph of the knee in an adult (left) and normal lateral radiograph of the knee in an adolescent (middle right). Note the thin soft tissue band (arrow) that represents a non-distended suprapatellar bursa that separates the suprapatellar and prefemoral fat pads. Also note the normal fragmentation of the tibial tuberosity in an adolescent. (Medial femoral condyle (1), lateral femoral condyle (2), medial tibial plateau (3), lateral tibial plateau (4), tibial spines (5), patella (6), fibula (7), femoral intercondylar notch (8), popliteal notch (9), patella tendon (10), tibial tuberosity (11), quadriceps tendon (12), suprapatellar fat pad (13), Hoffa's fat pad (14), prefemoral fat pad (15)).

ABCs systematic assessment

- Adequacy
- Alignment
- Bone
- Cartilage and joints
- Soft tissues

Radiographic projections of knee

Standard	Additional
• Anteroposterior	• Skyline
• Lateral	• Tunnel (or "notch")
	• Internal and external obliques

Adequacy

Anteroposterior and lateral projections are standard. A lateral radiograph should use a horizontal beam to detect a lipohaemarthrosis in patients who have experienced trauma. A skyline view allows assessment of the patellofemoral articulation. A tunnel or notch view is valuable to identify osteochondral fractures or intra-articular bodies. Oblique views in internal and external rotation allow further evaluation of tibial plateau fractures and of the proximal tibiofibular joint.

Radiographic interpretation

The horizontal lateral radiograph is evaluated first and the ABCs systematic assessment should start with the soft tissues.

Lateral radiographs

Soft tissues – Occasionally, the order of the ABCs systematic assessment is worth changing (not least for elbows and knees). Lateral radiographs of the knee are taken with a cross table horizontal beam, so it is useful to evaluate the soft tissues first for joint effusion and, particularly, for the presence of a lipohaemarthrosis (fat-fluid level).

Fluid within the knee joint distends the suprapatellar bursa, causing the prefemoral and suprapatellar fat pads to become separated by a soft tissue band. In the absence of a knee effusion, the band is <5 mm thick. With small effusions, the band is 5-10 mm thick, and large effusions further widen the bursa and may obliterate the adjacent fat pads, resulting in loss of distinction of the posterior border of the quadriceps tendon. Effusions may be the result of fractures, any form of internal derangement, infection, or arthritis.

Intra-articular fractures may result in release of marrow fat into the joint. On a horizontal beam lateral view, the fat will be seen to layer above the fluid. This fat-fluid level, or lipohaemarthrosis, occurs in around 35% of patients with intra-articular fractures (most commonly of the lateral tibial plateau) and is diagnostic of the presence of such a fracture, even if the fracture line itself cannot be seen. Detection of a lipohaemarthrosis itself is an indication for referral to orthopaedic surgeons and for further imaging (nowadays magnetic resonance imaging).

Alignment – The tibial plateau should align with the femoral condyles. Anterior tibial displacement can occur with rupture of the anterior cruciate ligament, while posterior displacement can occur with rupture of the posterior cruciate ligament.

On a lateral view with the knee in 20-30° flexion, the ratio of the patella tendon length to patella length should be in the range 0.8-1.2. A high riding patella (patella alta) may be a congenital variant or the result of rupture of the patella tendon. A low riding patella (patella baja) may be a congenital variant or the result of rupture of the quadriceps tendon.

Bone – The cortices of the femur, tibia, patella, and fibula should be smooth, with no disruption of the trabecular pattern within the bones. A careful search should be made for intra-articular bodies, which may represent fracture fragments.

Cartilage and joints – If the film is taken without obliquity, the patellofemoral and femorotibial joint spaces may be seen.

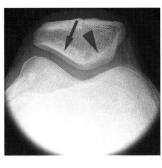

Normal skyline view of patella. The patella has a wider lateral (arrow) and narrower medial (arrowhead) articular facet for articulation with the anterior femoral condyles. Note the normal serrated appearance (known as patellar "teeth") of the anterior patellar cortex as a result of attachment of the extensor tendons.

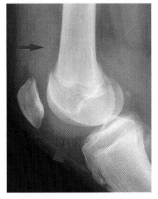

Lateral radiograph of the knee in a child after injury to anterior cruciate ligament. A large knee effusion causes distension of the suprapatellar bursa (arrow), with resulting wide separation of the suprapatellar and prefemoral fat pads. Fluid that indents the posterior aspect of the infrapatellar fat pad is also noted (arrowhead).

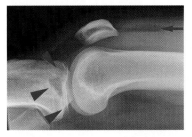

Horizontal beam lateral radiograph of the knee in patient with fracture of lateral tibial plateau. Large fat-fluid level (lipohaemarthrosis) in suprapatellar bursa (arrow) is consistent with presence of intra-articular fracture. Tibial plateau fracture is seen (arrowhead).

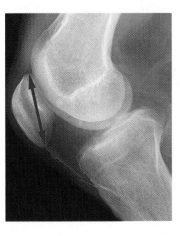

Normal lateral radiograph of the knee. The ratio of patella tendon length to patella length should be in range 0.8-1.2.

Anteroposterior radiographs

Interpretation of anteroposterior radiographs follows the same principles as for lateral radiographs, but joint effusions are not usually identifiable unless considerable fluid is present in the lateral joint recess. On this view, particular attention should be paid to identifying tibial plateau fractures, which may be seen as a subtle sclerotic line or a subtle step defect. A line through the lateral edge of the lateral femoral condyle (lateral tibial line) should run to the lateral edge of the lateral tibial plateau. The tibial plateau is not perfectly horizontal but slopes about 15° downwards from the anterior to the posterior cortex. In addition, the medial plateau is not flat but has a concave surface. The normal anteroposterior radiograph, therefore, may show parallel sclerotic lines at the tibial plateau, representing different portions of the plateau projected at slightly different levels on the film. The joint spaces in the medial and lateral compartments may be assessed on this view for height (reduced height may be the result of technical problems (knee flexion) or cartilage loss or arthritis) and for chondrocalcinosis (linear calcification within the cartilage, which may occur in patients with pseudogout or osteoarthritis).

Injuries

Distal femur

Femoral shaft fractures occur with considerable force. Anteroposterior and lateral views of the whole femur are essential to identify displacement and rotation.

Supracondylar fractures may have a variety of configurations. Evidence of intra-articular extension of the fracture line should be sought, as this necessitates open reduction and internal fixation. The distal fragment may be angulated by the pull of gastrocnemius, and displacement can result in popliteal artery injury. Occasionally, supracondylar fractures are associated with fracture dislocations of the hip or tibial shaft.

Femoral condylar fractures may show displacement or comminution and are often seen best with computed tomography. Shearing or rotatory forces directed at the articular surface of a femoral condyle may produce fractures, known as osteochondral fractures, through the cartilage and subchondral bone. These are often occult on conventional radiographs, but irregularity in the articular surface may be present and intra-articular fragments of bone may be seen.

Acute osteochondral fractures should be distinguished from osteochondritis dissecans. Osteochondritis dissecans occurs in adolescents at the lateral margin of the medial femoral condyle, and there may be a separated osteochondral fragment with sclerotic margins. The aetiology of this condition is controversial, but it may involve trauma.

Proximal tibia and fibula

Tibial plateau fractures occur most often in women >50 years, usually after twisting falls. Typically, valgus force is encountered, with impaction of the femoral condyle on the plateau, and involvement is confined to the lateral plateau in 75-80% of cases. Fewer than 25% of cases are the result of incidents between motor vehicles and pedestrians, and these typically result from the bumper of a car striking the knee. These fractures are often subtle, and anteroposterior and

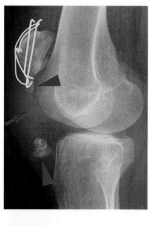

Lateral radiograph of the knee in a patient with patellar tendon rupture after repair of a patellar fracture. The patellar fracture was successfully repaired with two K wires and a tension band wire, as shown, but the patient suffered subsequent injury with rupture of the patellar tendon (arrow). Note the marked patellar alta and the soft tissue thickening at the site of the patellar tendon. Dystrophic ossification has developed within the proximal and distal portions of the disrupted tendon (arrowheads).

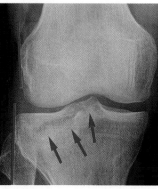

Anteroposterior radiograph of the knee in a patient with a fracture of the lateral tibial plateau. Lateral tibial line is abnormal, and fracture site is noted (arrow).

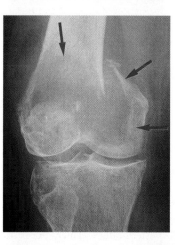

Anteroposterior radiograph of the knee in a patient with a supracondylar femoral fracture. Note: it is a pathological fracture that has occurred through a large lytic lesion (myeloma – arrows).

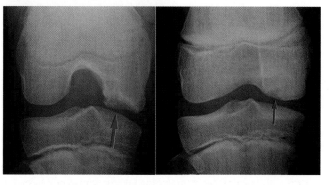

Notch (or tunnel) view (left) and anteroposterior view (right) of an adolescent with osteochondritis dissecans. There is an osteochondral defect (arrows) at the lateral aspect of the medial femoral condyle. Note that the defect is most clearly visualised on the notch view.

lateral radiographs need careful examination. Computed tomography is valuable, as the degree of depression of the fracture determines the need for surgery, and this is difficult to assess on conventional radiographs. Alternatively, magnetic resonance imaging may be used to assess these injuries; it also shows associated ligamentous and meniscal injuries, which are reported in 68-97% of cases.

Tibial stress fractures may be seen as transversely orientated sclerotic or lucent lines, with adjacent sclerosis in the medulla of the medial proximal tibial metaphysis extending to the cortex. The patient may show evidence of osteoporosis.

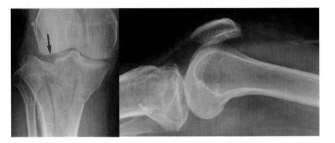

Anteroposterior radiograph of the knee in patient with comminuted tibial plateau fracture (left). Note the severe depression (arrow) and intra-articular fragments. Horizontal beam lateral radiograph of knee in same patient with tibial plateau fracture. Note the large lipohaemarthrosis (arrow) (right).

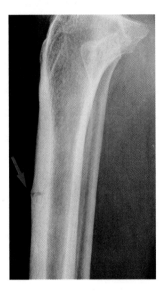

Lateral radiograph of the proximal tibia in a runner with a tibial stress fracture. A horizontal linear lucency (arrow) is seen at the anterior tibial cortex, with some surrounding cortical thickening.

Fibula head fractures may be isolated injuries that result from a direct blow, but they are associated most often with tibial plateau fractures. A fracture of the fibula neck or proximal shaft may suggest the presence of associated ankle joint injury (Maisonneuve). Proximal fibular fractures may be associated with common peroneal nerve injury.

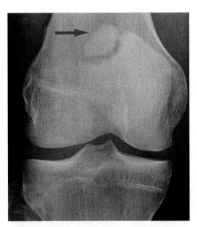

Anteroposterior radiograph of knee in patient with bipartite patella (arrow). This normal variant should not be confused with a fracture.

Patella

Patella fractures may be caused by a direct blow or by excessive quadriceps contraction during forced knee flexion. Fractures may be transverse, vertical, or comminuted, with or without displacement. These fractures can be difficult to detect on plain radiographs, but clinical examination should alert the doctor to the possibility, so most cases can be diagnosed after careful scrutiny of the films. A bipartite patella is a normal variant, which lies at the superolateral aspect of the patella, and which can be confused with a fracture.

Dislocation of the patella is almost always in the lateral direction and classically occurs in teenage girls. Dislocation is usually transient and presents with non-specific acute haemarthrosis. In many patients dislocation becomes recurrent. Radiographs after injury rarely show a dislocated patella, as the patella has usually been reduced by the time the radiograph has been taken. Usually, plain radiographs are normal apart from a joint effusion. A skyline view occasionally shows osteochondral injury, with fragments separated from the medial aspect of the patella or the anterior tip of the lateral femoral condyle, or both, as a result of impaction of the cortices at the time of transient dislocation.

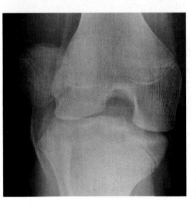

Anteroposterior radiograph of knee of an adolescent with lateral dislocation of patella.

Potential factors predisposing to lateral patellar dislocation

- Patella alta
- Shallow patellofemoral groove
- Genu valgum
- High "Q" angle

Knee dislocation

Dislocation of the knee is rare. Most commonly, anterior translation of the tibia on the femur is present, and the risk of popliteal artery and peroneal nerve injury is considerable. True knee dislocation is invariably associated with rupture of multiple ligaments, but plain radiographs are often misleading, with little or no abnormality visible, apart from a joint effusion. Magnetic resonance imaging should be performed to evaluate associated injuries.

Avulsion fractures and signs of ligamentous injury

Injury to ligamentous structures about the knee usually shows clinical signs of instability and a knee effusion. Avulsion fractures occasionally provide relatively specific evidence of particular ligamentous injuries.

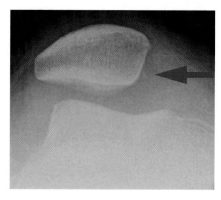

Skyline view of knee after relocation of patella. Note the patella remains laterally subluxed and a small bony avulsion fragment (arrow) is present medial to the patella.

Some signs of ligamentous injury visible on conventional radiographs of knee

Ligament	Sign of injury	Cause
Anterior cruciate ligament	Avulsion of anterior tibial eminence	• Avulsion of anterior cruciate ligament
	Segond fracture	• Lateral capsular ligament avulsion producing a small avulsion fragment at the lateral tibial plateau (>75% associated with injuries of anterior cruciate ligament)
	Deep notch	• Impaction of notch of lateral femoral condyle against posterior tibial plateau during injury of anterior cruciate ligament
Medial collateral ligament	Pellegrini-Stieda lesion	• Chronic recurrent injury of medial collateral ligament: shows linear calcification over the medial supracondylar edge
Lateral collateral ligament	Avulsion of fibular styloid process	• Avulsion of lateral collateral ligament and biceps femoris tendon
Quadriceps mechanism	Avulsion of superior or inferior patella pole	• Quadriceps contraction causing avulsion of distal quadriceps or proximal patella tendon
	Avulsion of tibial tuberosity*	• Quadriceps contraction causing avulsion of distal patella tendon

*This should be distinguished from Osgood-Schlatter's disease, a chronic condition occurring in adolescents characterised by anterior knee pain and fragmentation of the tibial tuberosity, with overlying soft tissue swelling

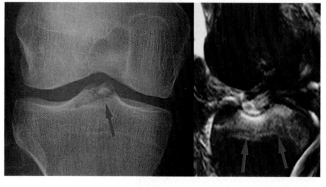

Patient with avulsion of anterior cruciate ligament. Anteroposterior radiograph of knee (left). Note avulsion of tibial spine (arrow). Sagittal magnetic resonance imaging scan of knee (right). Note avulsed anterior cruciate ligament with bony defect at site of insertion and extensive surrounding bright signal representing marrow oedema (arrows).

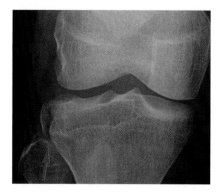

Anteroposterior radiograph of the knee in a patient with a Segond fracture. Note the small avulsion fragment at the lateral aspect of the lateral tibial plateau (arrow). This has a more than 75% association with anterior cruciate ligament injury.

Normal variants not to be confused with pathology

- Bipartite patella – secondary ossification centre at the supero-lateral patella
- Fabella – sesamoid bone in the lateral head of gastrocnemius
- Multiple ossification centres may occur at the apophysis for the tibial tuberosity
- Cortex of the posterosuperior femoral condyles may be irregular

KEY POINTS

- Diagnosis is strongly suspected on the basis of the clinical examination
- Unfortunately, clinical examination may be very difficult in an acutely injured knee. Plain radiographs can be misleading, as extensive derangement of the knee can occur with minimal or no radiographic findings
- Detection of a lipohaemarthrosis is an indication for further imaging and referral to an orthopaedic surgeon
- The threshold for requesting further imaging (magnetic resonance imaging, computed tomography, or ultrasonography) should be low

ABCs systematic assessment

Soft tissues
- Lipohaemarthrosis indicates intra-articular fracture

Alignment
- Anterior tibial displacement indicates anterior cruciate ligament rupture
- Posterior tibial displacement indicates posterior cruciate ligament rupture
- High riding patella (alta) indicates patella tendon rupture or congentital variant
- Low riding patella (baja) indicates quadriceps tendon rupture or congenital variant
- Femorotibial
- Patellofemoral

Bone
- Check femur, tibia, patella, fibula
- Tibial plateau should be evaluated carefully for subtle fractures
- Avulsion fragments may be a sign of ligament or tendon injury

Cartilage and joints
- Chondrocalcinosis indicates osteoarthritis, pseudogout
- Joint space narrowing indicates meniscal tear or cartilage loss

CHAPTER 8

Ankle

Paula McAlinden, James Teh

Trauma to the ankle is one of the most common reasons that people attend emergency departments. A spectrum of injuries can occur: from sprains through fractures to dislocations. The decision to obtain radiographs is made by careful clinical examination and knowledge of the mechanism of injury. The use of certain guidelines (such as the Ottawa rules) will exclude serious injuries while reducing unnecessary exposure of the patient to radiation. A higher index of suspicion is needed in elderly people, in whom a relatively minor injury can cause significant bony trauma.

Ottawa rules

- Bony tenderness at tip or posterior edge of distal 6 cm of tibia or fibula
- Bony tenderness of medial malleolus
- Tenderness at base of fifth metatarsal
- Unable to bear weight immediately or in emergency department

Anatomy

The ankle is a hinge joint made up of the medial malleolus of the tibia, the tibial plafond, and the lateral malleolus of the fibula, which articulates with the talar dome. The tibia and fibula form a ring (not dissimilar to that in the forearm) with the proximal and distal tibiofibular joints.

The bony structure of the ankle is stabilised by three main groups of ligaments:
- Medial collateral ligament complex (deltoid ligament)
- Lateral collateral ligament, which comprises anterior talofibular, posterior talofibular, and calcaneofibular ligaments
- Tibiofibular syndesmotic complex.

The talus articulates inferiorly with the calcaneus and anteriorly with the navicular. It is made up of a body, neck, and anterior process and has a fragile blood supply that extends through the ankle joint capsule, which means that fractures of the talar body may result in avascular necrosis.

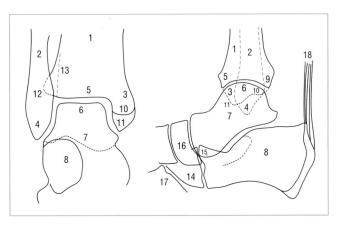

Anteroposterior views of ankle. Tibia (1), fibula (2), medial malleolus (3), lateral malleolus (4), plafond (5), dome (6), talus (7), calcaneum (8), posterior maleolus (9), anterior colliculus (10), posterior colliculus (11), anterior tubercle (12), peroneal groove (13), cuboid (14), anterior process (15), navicular (16), base of fifth metatarsal (17), achilles tendon (18).

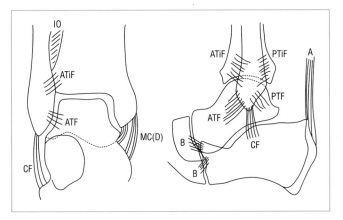

Ankle ligaments. A=Achilles tendon, ATiF=anterior tibiofibular, ATF=anterior talofibular, B=bifurcate, CF=calcaneofibular, D=deltoid, IO=interosseous, MC=medial collateral, PTiF=posterior tibiofibular, PTF=posterior talofibular.

Radiographic projections

Standard imaging of the ankle in the emergency department should include a lateral view and an anteroposterior view or anteroposterior view with 20° of internal rotation (mortice view). As a rule at least two views should be obtained for all cases of trauma because injuries are often missed on a single projection. Further imaging with ultrasonography, computed tomography, or magnetic resonance imaging may be needed to assess ligamentous injuries or complex fractures, but they should be performed only after consultation with a radiologist. The film exposure should allow visualisation of the soft tissues. In the anteroposterior view, the distal tibia and fibula should be seen to form the mortice around the talar dome. On the lateral view, the malleoli should overlap; the base of the fifth metatarsal should be included.

ABCs systematic assessment

- **Adequacy**
- **Alignment**
- **Bone**
- **Cartilage and joints**
- **Soft tissues**

Alignment

On the anteroposterior view, the uniform distance between the tibiotalar and fibulotalar joints should be <4 mm in adults. On the lateral view, the long axis of the tibia and fibula should overlap, and the axis should overlap the talar dome.

Bone

On the anteroposterior view, trace around the tibia, fibula, and talus – not forgetting their articular surfaces. On the lateral view, trace the cortical margins of the bones of the ankle joint, tibia, fibula, and talus, as well as the other bones on the radiograph, particularly the base of the fifth metatarsal and calcaneus. Abnormal steps in the cortex, lucent, or sclerotic lines sometimes indicate the presence of fractures. If no abnormality is seen on the anteroposterior view or on initial inspection of the lateral view, check the seven review areas (see line diagram opposite), in which subtle abnormalities can be missed.

Lateral malleolus – Oblique fractures can look normal on the anteroposterior view, so look through the tibia. Small flake fractures of the anterior margin of the tibial plafond can be easily overlooked on the lateral view. Small and even large posterior malleolus fractures can be difficult to detect and represent an unstable ankle injury. Flake fractures of the superior surface of the talus or navicula near the talonavicular joint can often be detected only with altering the imaging windows or magnification.

Calcaneal fractures usually occur as a result of direct impaction after a jump or fall from a height. They may be subtle. Compression fractures of the body of the calcaneus may extend to the subtalar joint. Stress fractures of the calcaneus usually occur in runners and may appear as a sclerotic linear band.

Fractures of the anterior process of the calcaneus (bifurcate ligament) are commonly missed. The fracture can be confirmed with an oblique projection.

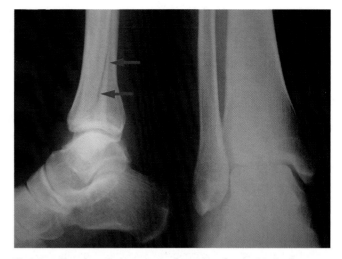

These two films show the importance of two views for trauma. On the anteroposterior view (left) there is no evidence of a fracture, but on the lateral view (right) there is clearly an oblique fracture of the fibular shaft (arrows).

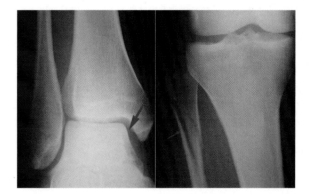

Loss of uniform joint space. Anteroposterior view (left) shows minimal widening of medial joint space (arrow), which is an important sign. Associated spiral fracture of proximal fibula is seen on the lateral radiograph (right) and is called a Maisonneuve fracture.

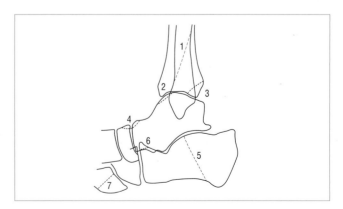

Review areas of ankle on lateral radiograph (lateral malleolus (1); tibial plafond (2); posterior malleolus (3); superior surface of the talus and navicular (4); calcaneus (5); anterior process of the calcaneus (bifurcate ligament) (6); base of the fifth metatarsal (7)).

Base of fifth metatarsal fracture is often missed, often because it is not seen on the lateral view and is on the edge of the film.

Cartilage and joints

The joint space should be the same on all sides of the ankle mortice on the anteroposterior and lateral views. The joint surface should be smooth, with no discontinuity. Small fractures, particularly of the talar dome, can have important consequences for a patient if missed.

Soft tissues

On the lateral view, the capsule of the ankle joint is distensible anteriorly and becomes prominent on the lateral radiograph as a teardrop shaped density when an effusion is present. This helpful sign should promote careful reinspection of the radiograph for occult fractures. On the anteroposterior view, swelling around the malleoli may indicate the site of injury.

Mechanisms of injury

Ankle injuries result from a combination of exaggerated normal movements that may be complicated by a twisting motion. The nature of the injury predicts the combination of bony and ligamentous injuries. For example, supination is a complex motion that consists of inversion and slight plantar flexion; pronation is a combination of eversion and dorsiflexion. Thus, these injuries can also involve the subtalar joint. Compression injuries (axial loading) result from direct landing onto the heel or foot. Such injuries are often predictable, with fractures of the calcaneus and talus being associated injuries.

Ankle sprains

Sprains usually occur after supination or inversion injuries. They most commonly involve the anterior talofibular ligament. Radiographs are not usually helpful. Ultrasonography or magnetic resonance imaging may be useful for further assessment of ligaments in selected patients. Clinically, severe ligamentous injuries may simulate fractures. Loss of alignment may be seen on plain radiographs.

Ankle fractures

Fractures of the ankle follow distinct patterns that depend on the mechanism of injury. This helps in the planning of surgical management. The Weber classification of ankle fractures is based on the position of the fibular fracture in relation to that of the inferior tibiofibular joint. The subtype of injury is related to the radiographic features, as well as the mechanism of injury and management needed. The classification also helps identify injuries that are most likely to involve the syndesmosis and thus cause instability of the ankle. These injuries are more likely to require surgical intervention.

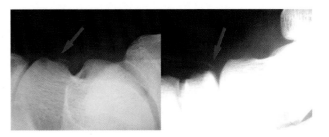

Fracture of the superior surface of the talus (arrow) (left) and fracture of the superior surface of the navicula (only visible with a bright light) (arrow) (right).

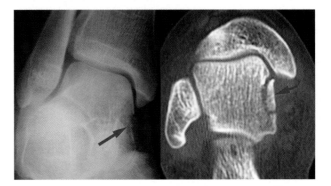

Small fractures of talar dome and talus can be difficult to diagnose (arrow) (left), but fracture of medial aspect of talus is easy to diagnose on computed tomography images (arrow) (right).

Normal ankle movements

- Dorsiflexion or plantar flexion – ankle joint
- Inversion or eversion – subtalar joint

West Point grading of ankle sprains

Criterion	Grade 1	Grade 2	Grade 3
Location of pain	Anterior talofibular ligament	Anterior talofibular ligament, and calcaneofibular ligament	Anterior talofibular ligament, calcaneofibular ligament, and posterior talofibular ligament
Oedema or bruising	Slight local	Moderate local	Substantial and diffuse
Weight bearing	Full or partial	Difficult without crutches	Impossible without pain
Ligament damage	Stretched	Partial tear	Complete tear
Instability	None	None or slight	Definite

Weber classification of ankle fractures

Type	Subtype	Mechanism	Syndesmosis	Imaging findings
A	1	Supination-adduction	Intact	Horizontal fibular fracture below ankle joint with associated oblique fracture of medial malleolus
	2			Intact fibula with disruption of lateral collateral ligament complex and medial malleolus fracture
B	1	Supination-external rotation	Intact	Spiral fracture of fibula and horizontal avulsion of medial malleolus and tear of tibiofibular ligaments
	2			Spiral fracture of fibula with rupture of deltoid ligament
C	1	Pronation-abduction	Disrupted	Fibular fracture above joint with rupture of tibiofibular ligaments and interosseus membrane and avulsion of medial malleolus
	2	Pronation-external rotation	Disrupted	Fibular fracture above joint with rupture of tibiofibular ligaments and interosseus membrane and rupture of deltoid ligaments

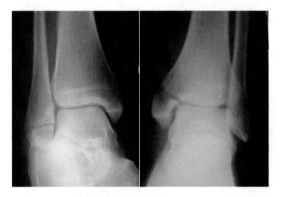

Weber A1: lateral malleolus fracture (left), and Weber A2: medial malleolus fracture (right).

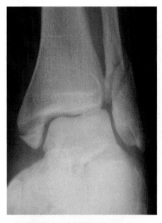

Weber B1: spiral fracture of fibula with horizontal medial malleolar fracture.

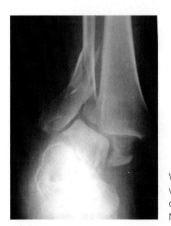

Weber C1: Fibular fracture above joint with avulsion of medial malleolus and disruption of tibiofibular ligaments. Note: tibiotalar dislocation.

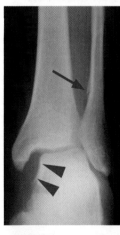

Weber C2: spiral fracture of fibula (arrow) with disruption of deltoid ligament (double arrowheads) (right).

Maisonneuve fracture

This is a variant of the pronation-external rotation fracture (Weber C2). A medial malleolus fracture is seen in the anteroposterior view; however, the fibular fracture is in the proximal end. Without careful examination of the proximal fibula in patients with fractures of the medial malleolus, these injuries may be missed. If the presence of a Maisonneuve fracture is suspected, a full length radiograph of the tibia and fibula should be obtained.

Trimalleolar

These fractures are caused by severe forces of abduction or external rotation. The fracture is made up of fractures of the medial, lateral, and posterior malleoli. The fracture is often associated with an

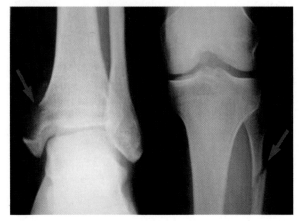

Maisonneuve fractures – medial malleolus fracture (arrow) (left) and proximal fibular fracture (right).

unstable ankle and may need surgical fixation, particularly if more than one-third of the articular surface of the tibia is involved.

Pylon

A pylon is an architectural term for a stone archway, which has been likened to the appearance of the ankle mortice. These fractures occur after axial compression injuries. The talus is driven upwards into the mortice with enough force to cause comminution of the tibial plafond and a fracture of the distal tibia above the ankle joint. Imaging with computed tomography is often used to assess the degree of comminution and the relation of fragments to the articulating surface. Almost invariably, these patients need operative management.

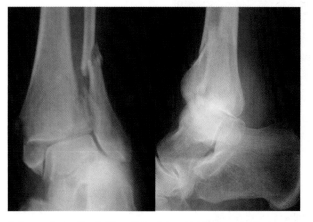

Anteroposterior view (left) and lateral view (right) of a pylon fracture.

Ankle dislocation

Ankle dislocation occurs as a result of substantial force to the joint leading to loss of apposition of the articular surfaces. Invariably there are associated fractures. The most common pattern of injury is posterior dislocation with the talus being driven posteriorly with respect to the tibia. This is accompanied by a disruption of the tibiofibular syndesmosis or a fracture of the lateral malleolus. Lateral dislocations may occur in association with fractures of the malleoli. As with any dislocation, neurovascular injury is the main concern. Avascular necrosis of the talus may occur if joint reduction is delayed.

Fractures involving the growth plate

Tillaux – This fracture is characterised by avulsion of the distal end of the tibia medially. The medial distal tibia is avulsed. In children, it is called a juvenile Tillaux and constitutes a Salter-Harris III fracture. The mechanism of injury is abduction and external rotation, and the fracture is thought to result from a tear of the anterior inferior tibiofibular ligament. The extent of the fracture is clearly defined in computed tomography imaging scans.

Triplane – This complex fracture is an injury seen in children. As its name suggests, the fracture runs in the coronal and sagittal plane, with the axial plane running through the distal epiphysis. These fractures can be subtle, but suspicion should be raised if the anteroposterior view shows a vertical fracture of the epiphysis. Careful inspection of the lateral view will often show the diaphyseal component, but unfortunately it is often normal. Computed tomography imaging of these fractures is invaluable in surgical planning.

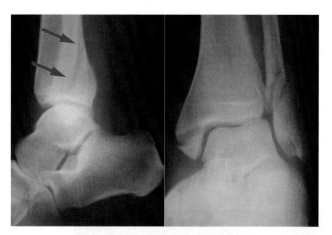

Lateral view of posterior malleolar fracture (arrow) (left) and anteroposterior view of medial and lateral malleolar fractures (right).

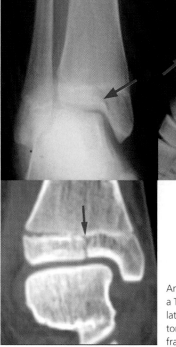

Ankle dislocation – large displaced posterior malleolar fracture (arrow) with a posterior dislocation of talus (arrowhead).

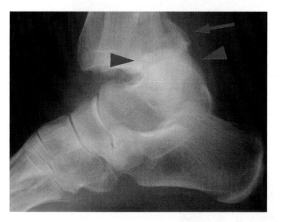

Anteroposterior view of ankle with a Tillaux fracture (top left) and lateral view (top right). Computed tomography scan (left) shows Tillaux fracture.

Talar fractures

Osteochondral fractures of the talus occur as the result of impaction of the talar dome against the tibial plafond. If they are unstable, they may result in a loose body within the joint.

Talar neck fractures are important because of the risk of ischaemic necrosis of the talus. The degree of displacement of the fracture indicates the probability of this serious complication developing. The most widely used classification is the Hawkins classification, which relates displacement of the fracture with risk of ischaemic necrosis.

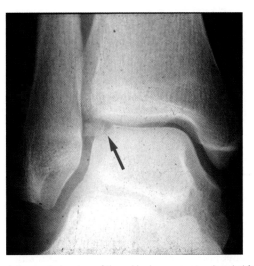

Anteroposterior view of the ankle shows an osteochondral fracture of the talar dome (arrow).

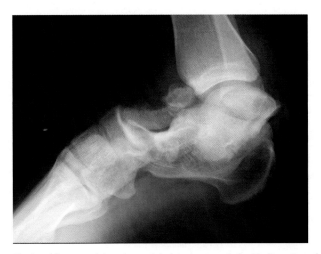

Displaced fracture of the talar neck (aviator's astragalus) with disruption of the talonavicular and subtalar joints (Hawkins IV).

Hawkins classification of talar neck fractures

- I – undisplaced fracture (0-10% risk)
- II – slightly displaced (about a 40% risk)
- III – severe displacement with disruption of subtalar and tibiotalar joint (>70%)
- IV – displaced fracture with disruption of talonavicular joint (high risk)

Catches to avoid

Fractures may be simulated by accessory ossicles. These developmental abnormalities can often be mistaken for avulsion injuries. They are usually rounded, with a well corticated margin, whereas avulsion injuries have a sharp margin, are not well corticated, and fit like pieces in a jigsaw puzzle to the adjacent bone.

KEY POINTS

- Imaging is based on clinical presentation and mechanism of injury
- Ankle and foot injuries can occur simultaneously. Subtle injuries can be diagnosed on the lateral radiograph
- Use the ABCs systematic assessment
- Substantial soft tissue injuries can occur with normal radiographs

ABCs systematic assessment

Alignment
- There should be a uniform joint space in the tibiotalar and talofibular joints
- The fibula should overlap the talar dome on the lateral view

Bone
- Check distal fibula for an avulsion
- Check the cortical outline of the tibia and fibula
- Check the cortical outline of the talus

Review areas
- Check the fibular shaft is intact on the lateral view
- Check the talar dome for fractures
- Check that the posterior malleolus is intact
- Check the superior talonavicular joint on the lateral view
- Check the posterior process of the calcaneus
- Check the anterior process of the calcaneus is intact
- Check the base of the fifth metatarsal is intact

Cartilage and joints
- Joint space should be uniform

Soft tissues
- Soft tissue swelling around the malleoli may indicate the site of injury
- Displacement of the fat pad at the anterior joint line on the lateral view may indicate an effusion which should prompt a search for a fracture

CHAPTER 9

Foot

Peter Renton, Muaaze Ahmad, Otto Chan

Injuries of the feet often result in a request for radiographs of the ankle and foot. Clinically, it should be possible to distinguish which area has been injured, and imaging of both is rarely needed. Injuries to the feet, however, often masquerade as ankle injuries. Often the patient cannot remember the exact nature of the injury – except for a twisting injury of the ankle and foot. The clinical history can be useful in predicting injuries. Injuries to the feet can occur from various mechanisms.

Anatomy

The foot is a complex structure of interdependent bones designed for weightbearing and movement. It can be divided into the forefoot, midfoot, and hindfoot. The joints are complex, but the articular surfaces are parallel and the joint spaces equidistant and symmetrical. Loss of articular parallelism and alteration of joint space width is always abnormal.

Plain radiography

Site of injury	Projection
Hindfoot	Lateral
	Oblique
	Axial (Harris)
Forefoot and midfoot	Anteroposterior
	Oblique
	Lateral
Phalanges	Anteroposterior
	Oblique
	Elevated lateral of toe

Mechanism of injury

- Objects falling onto feet – forefoot injuries
- Kicking objects – big toe injuries
- Hitting objects barefoot – little toe fractures and dislocations
- Landing from a height (falls) – calcaneal fractures
- Twisting ankle – base of fifth metacarpal avulsion fractures
- Overuse – stress fractures

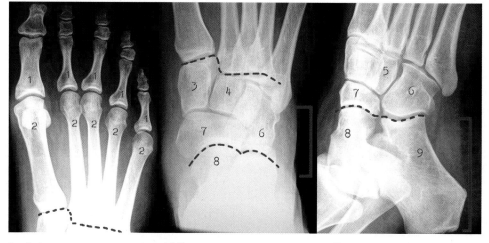

Forefoot   Midfoot   Hindfoot

Forefoot: Phalanges (1), Metatarsals (2). Midfoot: Cuneiforms – Medial (3), Middle (4), Lateral (5) – Cuboid (6), Navicula (7). Hindfoot: Talus (8), Calcaneum (9).

Normal variants

Plain films may show variation from the normal anatomy because of the presence of sesamoids, fused or partly fused bones, or accessory ossification centres. Although these are normal variants, they can also be the sites of pathology. Commonly occurring ossicles are the os tibiale externum (medial to the navicular), os trigonum (posterior to the talus), and os peroneum (adjacent to the cuboid). Accessory ossicles are also often found beneath the malleoli. Secondary ossification centres can occur anywhere, but they are particularly common in the feet. There are two sesamoids on the big toe. None of these normal variants should be confused with fractures.

ABCs systematic assessment

- **A**dequacy, alignment
- **B**one
- **C**artilage and joints
- **S**oft tissues

Adequacy

Not all bones and joints will be seen clearly on one view, so multiple views will be needed. Some injuries are visualised poorly on plain radiography, and computed tomography or other types of imaging may be needed.

Other types of imaging

Type	Feature
Ultrasonography	Used to assess soft tissues, muscles, tendons, and ligaments
	Effusions and other fluid collections can be seen and aspirated
	Very dependent on the operator
Computed tomography	Axial slices obtained with multiplanar reconstruction
	Good for looking at bones, bone bars, and fractures
Magnetic resonance imaging	Highly sensitive and specific
	Shows pathology in bones, joints, and soft tissues
	Multiplanar imaging, usually axial, sagittal, and coronal
Isotopes	Increase of isotope uptake in bones is a non-specific, highly sensitive indicator of disease

Alignment

On plain x rays of the lateral view, the superior surfaces of the talus, navicular, medial cuneiform, and first metatarsal lie in a straight line. Böhler's angle lies between the plane of the posterosuperior and anterosuperior surfaces of the calcaneus and measures 28-40° in normal feet. Flattening of the angle (<28°) follows calcaneal compression with trauma.

The midtarsal joint separates the talus and calcaneus from the navicular and cuboid. This curvilinear joint line resembles a wave (or cyma). An intact cyma line shows integrity of the midtarsal joints.

Beneath the talus lie the posterior subtalar joint, sinus tarsi, and middle subtalar joint. These are seen on lateral, oblique, and axial images but are best visualised with computed tomography and magnetic resonance imaging. The cyma line is also seen at the midtarsal joint on the anteroposterior and oblique views.

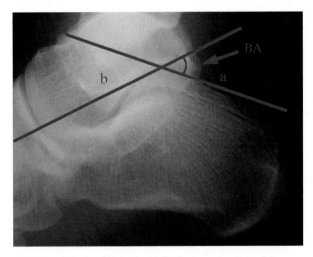

Common accessory ossicles. Os trigonum (1), os supratalare (2), os supranaviculare (3), os calcaneum secundarius (4), os peroneum (5), os vesalaneum (6), os tibiale externum (7), os intercuneiforme (8), os intermetatarseum (9).

Böhler's angle (BA), which is 28-40°, lies between the plane of the posterosuperior (a) and anterosuperior (b) surfaces of the calcaneum.

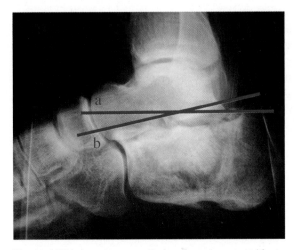

Disrupted Böhler's angle as a result of a calcaneal commuted fracture.

The midfoot articulates with the forefoot. The tarsometatarsal joint must be evaluated carefully, as subluxations and dislocations of this region can be subtle and easily missed, leading to disastrous consequences.

- Line 1 – In the anteroposterior view of the foot, the medial aspect of the second metatarsal should align with the medial aspect of the middle cuneiform.
- Line 2 – On the oblique view of the foot, the medial aspect of the third metatarsal should align with the medial aspect of the lateral cuneiform.
- Line 3 – Also on the oblique view, the medial aspect of the fourth metatarsal should align with the medial aspect of the cuboid.

The appearance and alignment of the toes are variable, and any suspicious areas on radiographs should be compared with clinical findings.

Bone

Trace the outlines of all the bones in a systematic order, particularly the cortical margins of the bones affected by the injury. The correct views must be obtained. In particular, check the anterior process of the calcaneum, which is commonly avulsed with inversion ankle injuries by the bifurcate ligament. This ligament has two limbs: one attaches to the navicular and the other to the cuboid.

Cartilage and joints

In the feet, subluxations and dislocations can be very subtle on plain radiographs, and it is critical that they are not missed.

Soft tissues

On plain radiographs, the soft tissues should be inspected first. The absence of soft tissue swelling usually rules out underlying pathology; conversely, soft tissue swelling may indicate local underlying disease. The achilles tendon and plantar fascia, as well as joint capsules, may also be seen on plain films, because they are surrounded by, and are denser than, adjacent fat.

Calcaneal injuries

Fractures in adults usually result from falls from a height and are associated with lumbar vertebral body compression fractures. In patients who have fallen from a height and have sustained compression fractures of the calcaneum, the threshold for taking radiographs of the spine, pelvis, and whole limb and the opposite calcaneum should be low.

Seventy-five per cent of adult calcaneal fractures involve the main part of the body and the subtalar joints. About half show serious displacement. In children, most calcaneal fractures are peripheral or extra-articular.

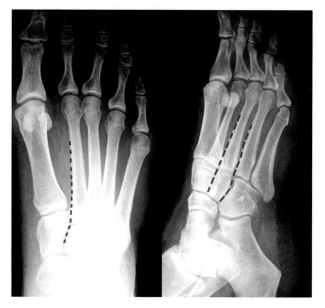

Anteroposterior and oblique radiographs of foot showing lines 1 (left), 2, and 3 (right).

Calcaneal fractures

- Body and subtalar joint
- Extra-articular
  Anterior process
  Tuberosity
  Posterior aspect (beak)
- Calcaneus (60% of fractures of the foot)

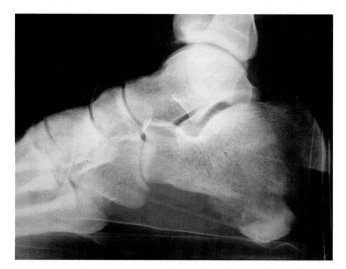

Lateral radiograph of foot showing calcaneal compression fracture.

Fractures through the body of the calcaneus are often comminuted and involve the sustentaculotalar joints and sustentaculum tali. Images from computed tomography scanning with multiplanar and three dimensional reconstruction should always be done to assess the true extent of injury and to plan surgery. Computed tomography images show the direction of fracture lines and the involvement of subtalar joint facets. Vertical compression is associated with lateral and medial displacement of the fracture parts. Displacement of the sustentaculum may be seen.

Fractures of the subtalar joints may result in articular incongruity and subsequent osteoarthritis. Compression of the superior surface of the calcaneus leads to a diminution of Böhler's angle

Twenty-five per cent of calcaneal fractures in adults are extra-articular, involving the anterior process, tuberosity, or posterior aspect of the bone (beak). The "beak fracture" shows elevation of the posterosuperior surface of the calcaneus. The achilles tendon may avulse the bone at its insertion.

Fractures of the apophysis occur in children, but the normal apophysis may have a fragmented or sclerotic appearance before fusion. Trauma will be associated with local soft tissue swelling and pain.

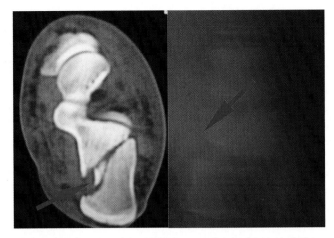

Axial computed tomography scan of calcaneum showing a comminuted fracture (arrow) (left) and anteroposterior view of associated lumbar spine compression burst fracture (right).

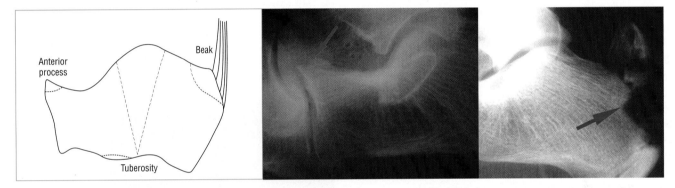

Extra-articular calcaneal fracture lines (left), anterior process fracture (arrow) (middle), and beak fracture (right).

Stress fractures of the calcaneus and foot

These fractures appear as sclerotic lines and can have subtle or even normal appearances on plain radiographs. They are relatively common and may occur in the young and in soldiers (through normal bone), and in older people, often through osteoporotic bone (in older women after minimal force). Patients have pain and tenderness in the foot, which is worse on exercise and relieved with rest. If such an injury is suspected but images from plain radiography are normal, further imaging with isotope computed tomography or magnetic resonance imaging should be obtained.

Talus

Fractures of the talus mainly occur in adults and are generally uncommon. Chip or avulsion fractures are the most frequent fractures (50%) and fractures of the talar neck are the next most common (30%).

Talar neck fractures (the aviator's astragalus) result from high velocity impaction and may lead to avascular necrosis of the body of the talus. Plain radiographs and computed tomography images show changes of avascular necrosis at 6-8 weeks. The talar dome shows flattening and sclerosis. Long term follow-up is indicated, as

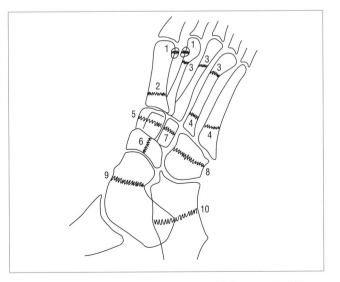

Stress fractures of foot and calcaneum. Sesamoids (1); first metatarsal (2), neck of second to fourth metatarsals (3), base of fourth and fifth metatarsal (4), medial cuneiform (5), navicula (6), lateral cuneiform (7), cuboid (8), talus (9), calcaneum (10).

changes of avascular necrosis may be delayed. Magnetic resonance imaging is much more sensitive at detecting such fractures and bone marrow oedema. Talar neck fractures also result in delayed or non-union and in secondary osteoarthritis.

Talar and subtalar dislocations

Most of these dislocations are associated with talar fractures. Those without fractures must involve simultaneous dislocation of the talonavicular joint. Pure talar dislocation is seen rarely but is very disabling and involves the ankle, subtalar, and talonavicular joints. Most subtalar dislocations are reduced easily and should be reduced if detected clinically. Subluxations can be very subtle, however, and unless there is meticulous evaluation of the subtalar joint, these dislocations are often missed. The key is to evaluate the alignment of the talonavicular and calcaneocuboid joints by confirming an intact cyma line.

Computed tomography scanning should always be done as osteochondral fractures are common. These fractures may prevent reduction and may lie within the joints, resulting in premature osteoarthritis.

Osteochondral fractures of the talar dome

These may be seen on plain films but are best visualised in images from computed tomography or magnetic resonance imaging. They typically occur on the anterolateral and posteromedial aspects of the talar dome. The lateral lesions in particular result in pain and locking.

Navicular, cuboid and cuneiform fractures

Isolated fractures of these bones are relatively rare. Avulsion fractures of the navicular, at the talonavicular joint superiorly or the medial aspect by the posterior tibialis tendon, are the most common.

Tarsometatarsal joints (Lisfranc's joints)

A transverse ligament connects the bases of the second to fifth metatarsals, but no such ligament exists medially between the first and second metatarsals. This arrangement potentiates lateral displacement of the second to fifth metatarsals.

Lisfranc's fracture-dislocation

This is an uncommon but important injury, in which the foot is forced into plantar flexion alone or is also rotated. Different patterns of dislocation are seen at the tarsometatarsal joints, and these are best seen with plain films.

Fractures may result from crush injuries, which produce a comminuted or transverse fracture, while indirect trauma from a twist can result in spiral fractures. Shortening of the metatarsal results, and there is subsequent alteration of weightbearing stresses.

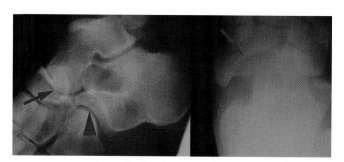

Fracture of head and neck of talus with dislocated talonavicular joint (arrow). Note: associated fracture of the anterior process of the calcaneum (arrowhead).

Patterns of Lisfranc's fracture-dislocation

- Hallux metatarsal may dislocate medially (divergent)
- Four lateral metatarsals may dislocate laterally
  Associated with fracture of base of second metatarsal, which is proximal to the other metatarsal bases
  Fracture of second metatarsal base occurs because of its proximal recession
  Laterally subluxed fourth and fifth metatarsal bases lie lateral to cuboid
- Dorsal and lateral dislocation of the lateral four, or all, metatarsals (homolateral)
- Proximal separation of the medial and middle cuneiforms

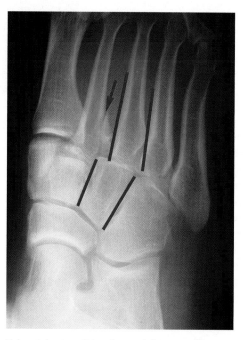

Lisfranc's fracture-dislocation: malalignment of lines 2 and 3. Also associated with a fracture at the base of the second metatarsal (arrow).

Fracture of the base of the fifth metatarsal

The normal apophysis at the base of the fifth metatarsal may remain unfused and should not be confused with a fracture. Its margins are well defined and corticated, and alignment of the growth plate is sagittal. Local fractures tend to be oblique or transverse and associated with overlying soft tissue swelling. The fracture itself will not be corticated internally. Transverse fractures, especially in young athletic people, have a high incidence of non-union.

Robert Jones described a fracture he sustained while dancing. It was about 2 cm distal to the metatarsal base, which is not the avulsion lesion of the tuberosity at the base of the fifth metatarsal caused by the tendon of peroneus brevis, although both occur after inversion injuries to the ankle. Robert Jones' fracture may undergo delayed or non-union and may need internal fixation.

Phalanges

Fractures to the phalanges usually result from direct trauma – for example, from crush injuries. Always look at adjacent phalanges and toes.

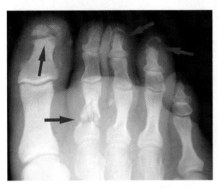

Multiple crush fractures of toes (arrows).

Other stress lesions in the foot

Stress fractures often occur at the second and third metatarsal shafts and are seen in new army recruits, joggers, and dancers. Stress lesions or osteochondritic changes also occur in the hallux sesamoids, (second metatarsal head – Freiberg's disease), and os trigonum in footballers and ballet dancers.

Avascular necrosis of the navicular (Köhler's disease) may be ischaemic in origin. Sever's disease (osteochondritis of the posterior calcaneal apophysis) may be a traction phenomenon, but sclerosis and fragmentation of the apophysis are normal variants.

KEY POINTS

- Considerable overlap is seen in ankle and foot injuries. Alignment must be checked meticulously as serious injuries can be subtle
- Request and obtain correct views
- The threshold for requesting computed tomography, magnetic resonance imaging, and isotopes should be low
- Stress fractures in the foot are common and can be subtle

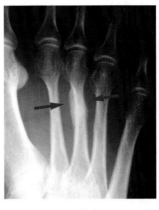

Stress fracture of third metatarsal (arrows).

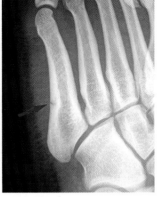

Stress fracture of fifth metatarsal (arrow).

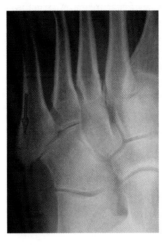

Transverse fracture of base of fifth metatarsal (arrow).

ABCs systematic assessment

Alignment

- Check talonavicular joint is intact to exclude a pure talus dislocation
- Make sure the cyma line is intact to exclude a midtarsal dislocation
- Carefully check lines 1-3 to exclude a Lisfranc's injury

Bone

- Follow contour of talar dome to exclude an osteochondrial fracture
- Fractures of the calcaneum can be subtle. Look for a disruption of the trabelulae and subtle sclerotic or lucent lines
- Check for flake fractures of the superior surface of the navicular on the lateral ankle view
- Fractures of the cuboid and cuneiform are uncommon
- Do not confuse apophysis with fracture of fifth metatarsal
- Check all phalanges in crush injuries using a bright light

Cartilage and joints

- Look for widened joint space. A disrupted cyma line indicates midtarsal dislocation
- Disrupted lines 1-3 indicate a Lisfranc's injury
- Check cyma sign and Lisfranc's joint

Soft tissues

- Swelling indicates site of injury

CHAPTER 10

Chest

Ali Naraghi, Otto Chan

Chest radiographs are among the most commonly requested radiological investigations in emergency departments. A structured systematic assessment is needed to ensure that potentially serious conditions are not overlooked, particularly because a wide variety of conditions can be encountered. Many (but by no means all) common and acute life threatening conditions are covered in this chapter. Successful interpretation of a chest radiograph needs an understanding of the appearance of a normal chest radiograph.

Chest radiographs

Anteroposterior view (low kV)
- Standard view for patients in emergency departments and intensive care units, for taking portable radiographs, and for patients who are supine
- Usually erect but can be supine
- Patient often rotated
- Patient often unable to take a good breath
- Good for evaluation of skeleton
- Reasonable for lung pathology
- Not good for evaluating mediastinum

Posteroanterior view (high kV)
- Standard projection
- Best technique
- Excellent for lungs and mediastinum
- Poor for evaluation of skeleton
- Cannot be done in patients with trauma and those who are supine

Anatomy

The posteroanterior view is taken with the patient facing the film and with the x ray tube behind the patient, usually in a dedicated chest room with a side marker fixed to the machine. This view is taken in the erect position in full inspiration. It shows the cardiomediastinal contour with lower magnification than the anteroposterior view. It also gives a clearer view of the lungs, because the scapulae are projected outside the lungs.

The anteroposterior view is performed when a patient cannot walk, is having a portable film, or is unconscious. In this view (low kV) the bones are seen clearly, but the lungs are not as well visualised. The patient may be rotated, the film exposure may be incorrect, and the patient could have taken a poor inspiration. The scapulae usually project over the lateral aspect of the lungs.

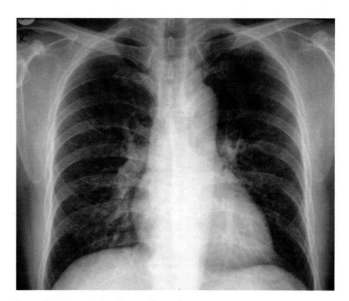

Normal posteroanterior chest radiograph.

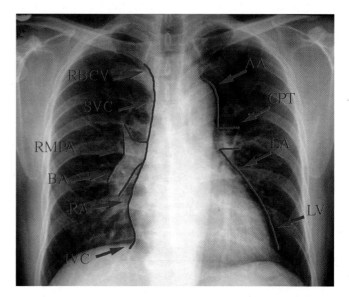

Normal posteroanterior chest radiograph (AA=arch of aorta, BA=basal artery, CPT=common pulmonary trunk, IVC=inferior vena cava, LA=left atrium, LV=left ventricle, RA=right atrium, RBCV= right brachiocephalic vein, RMPA=right main pulmonary artery, SVC=superior vena cava).

The right side of the mediastinum (superior to inferior) consists of the right brachiocephalic vein, superior vena cava, and right atrium. The left mediastinal border (superior to inferior) comprises the left subclavian artery, aortic arch, main pulmonary artery, left atrial appendage, and left ventricle. The cardiophrenic fat pads may be seen as prominent opacities that simulate a mass lesion or area of consolidation.

The right lung consists of three lobes (upper, middle, and lower lobes) separated by horizontal and oblique fissures. The left lung comprises two lobes (upper and lower lobes) separated by the oblique fissure. On a normal posteroanterior chest radiograph only the horizontal fissure is seen, whereas on lateral chest radiographs, the horizontal and oblique fissures are seen. Occasionally, other accessory fissures, such as the azygos fissure may be seen.

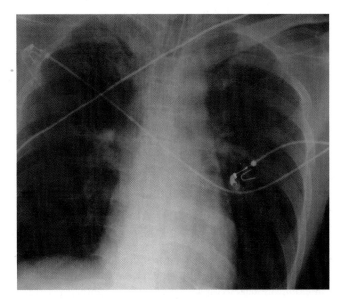

Normal anteroposterior chest radiograph.

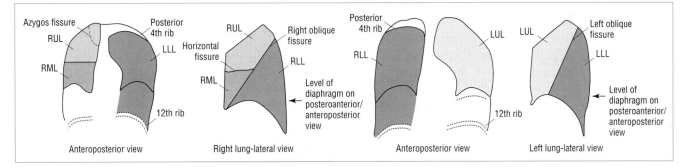

Lung fissures and lobes (LLL= left lower lobe, LUL=left upper lobe, RML= right middle lobe, RLL=right lower lobe, RUL=right upper lobe).

Lungs are divided on the frontal chest radiographs into three zones: upper zone (above the lower border of the anterior aspect of the second rib), mid zone (between the anterior aspects of the second and fourth ribs), and lower zone (below the lower border of the fourth rib anteriorly to the diaphragm). This has no correlation to the lobes, but is used to describe the position of any abnormality seen on frontal chest radiographs. One third of the lungs lies below the level of the diaphragm. The diaphragm is attached onto the twelfth rib inferiorly.

The posterior ribs lie horizontally and arise from the spine. The anterior ribs tend to slope inferiorly and anteriorly, and they fade medially (the anterior aspect of the ribs is joined to the sternum by cartilage, hence they fade anteriorly).

Initially, chest radiographs should be assessed for life threatening acute emergencies, and then the more standard systematic review of chest radiographs can be performed. The ABCs systematic assessment described in this chapter can be used for interpretation of all chest radiographs – whether on posteroanterior or anteroposterior views taken supine or erect or in patients with acute and non-acute conditions.

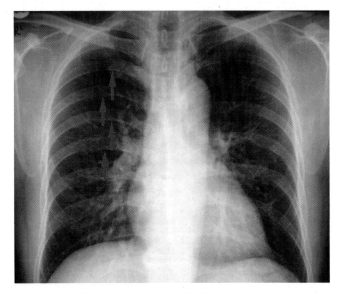

Posterior (arrows) and anterior (arrowheads) ribs.

ABCs systematic assessment

- **A**dequacy, **a**irways, **a**ll lines
- **B**reathing
- **C**irculation
- **D**iaphragm
- **E**dges
- **S**keleton, **s**oft tissues

Adequacy

Check these items when you review chest radiographs.
- Name marker: check the patient's name
- Side marker: ensure you know which side is which
- Correct area: film should include an area from the lung apices to the costophrenic angles
- Inspiration: at least five anterior ribs should be seen above the midpoint of the hemidiaphragms. Visualisation of fewer than five anterior ribs suggests the patient took a poor breath
- Rotation: medial ends of the clavicles should be equidistant from the spinous process of the vertebra at that level. The patient should be straight enough so that rotation does not interfere with interpretation of the film
- Exposure: on a correctly exposed film, the lower thoracic vertebrae (T8/T9 disc) and the left lower lobe pulmonary vessels should be visible through the cardiac silhouette.

Airways

Trachea

The trachea should be central above the manubrium but deviates slightly to the right below this. Check the position of the endotracheal tube.

Bronchi

Any deviation not accounted for by rotation suggests ipsilateral collapse, scarring, fibrosis, or surgery on the same side. Contralateral shift is the result of a mass effect: tension pneumothorax, haemothorax, or large effusion. The right mainstem bronchus should have a more vertical alignment than the left main bronchus. Exclude teeth and foreign bodies.

All lines

Endotracheal tube

The tip of the endotracheal tube should be at the level of the aortic arch or at least 3.5-5.5 cm above the carina. This is because the film is exposed with the neck in extension. Having the tip of the endotracheal tube at least 3.5 cm above the carina ensures that the tube does not extend past the carina if the neck is flexed. If the endotracheal tube tip is too low, it is likely to obstruct the left lower lobe or the right upper lobe bronchi and cause the lung to collapse. Also check the position of the nasogastric tube on the chest radiograph.

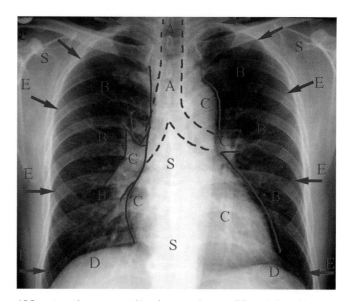

ABCs systematic assessment (A=adequacy, airways, all lines; B=breathing; C=circulation; D=diaphragm; E=edges; S=skeleton, soft tissues).

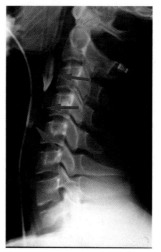

Several teeth in airway (arrows).

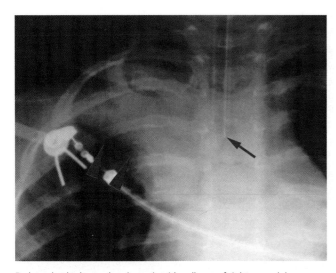

Endotracheal tube too low (arrow), with collapse of right upper lobe (arrowheads).

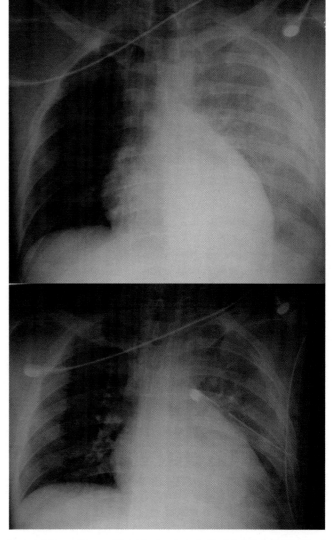

Large left haemothorax with tracheal and mediastinal deviation to right (top) and after chest drain insertion (bottom). Note: trachea and mediastinum have shifted back to normal position (bottom).

Venous catheters

Intravenous central lines should not be kinked and should follow the smooth curve of the vessels. The tip of the line should be straight because a curvature suggests that the tip is impinging on the vessel wall.

Chest drains

Chest drains have a radio-opaque line within their wall. A break in this radio-opaque line indicates the site of the last hole in the tube, and it is essential to ensure that this hole lies within the thoracic cavity. A chest drain inserted in the right midaxillary line, which extends to the right hilum, will probably be located within the horizontal fissure.

Breathing

Exclude a tension pneumothorax or haemothorax and check the ribs for fractures and radiologic flail segments. Confirm that the lungs are well aerated and clear. Check the position of chest drains and intravenous access lines. Assess and interpret lung abnormalities.

Circulation (mediastinum, hila, and pulmonary vasculature)

Check the following items when reviewing patients' chest radiographs.
- Heart size
- Mediastinal position: one third to the right, two thirds to the left of the midline
- Mediastinal contour: clearly defined margins, especially aortic contour

Measurement of heart size

Posteroanterior chest radiograph
- Transverse cardiac diameter 1 cm greater than the value for a posteroanterior radiograph if there is no rotation
- Cardiothoracic ratio <0.5

Anteroposterior chest radiograph
- Transverse cardiac diameter 1 cm, ignore if there is no rotation
- Cardiothoracic ratio <0.6 (good inspiration and no rotation)

- Widening of mediastinum in trauma indicates mediastinal haematoma and a traumatic aortic injury should be excluded with computed tomography. In the absence of trauma, it usually indicates a mass or lymphadenopathy
- Hila: evaluate size, shape, and position. Basal artery size is 16 mm in men and 15 mm in women. It should taper and the right hilum is usually lower or, rarely, the same level as the left hilum. Enlargement of one hilum usually indicates a mass or lymphadenopathy. Enlargement of both hila is either the result of lymphadenopathy or is vascular in nature.
- Lung vessel pattern: In a normal x ray there should be an even distribution and lower zone vessels should be larger than upper.

Diaphragm

Hemidiaphragms should have a sharp outline throughout their course. Loss of this outline indicates a pathological process in the lower lobe. The right hemidiaphragm normally lies 2.5 cm above the left hemidiaphragm. The area below the diaphragms should be assessed for free intraperitoneal air or abnormal areas of calcification.

Edges (pleura)

The costophrenic angles normally form an acute angle. Obliteration of this angle is seen in the presence of pleural fluid or thickening. Pleura are not normally seen on a chest radiograph. Visualisation of the pleura indicates the presence of air in the pleural cavity (pneumothorax).

Skeleton

Bones should be assessed for fractures or focal lesions such as metastatic deposits. In addition, the vertebrae can be assessed through the cardiac silhouette on a correctly exposed film. Bilateral paravertebral stripes are present: the left paravertebral stripe should measure <1 cm and the right paravertebral stripe should be <3 mm. These may become displaced by paravertebral haematomas secondary to the vertebral fractures.

Soft tissues

Soft tissues should be examined with regard to the presence of air (surgical emphysema) and foreign bodies. Check that the breasts are present.

Systematic review of the lungs

This chapter gives a brief summary of some, but not all, traumatic and non-traumatic conditions.

Compare the two lungs, particularly for volume and transradiancy. A hyperlucent lung may result from rotation of the patient, mastectomy, bronchial obstruction with air trapping, compensatory

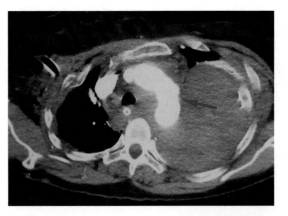

Computed tomography image of traumatic aortic injury (arrow).

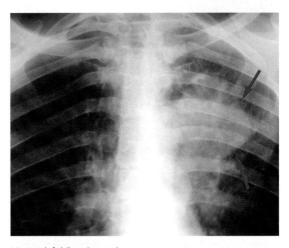

Mass at left hilum (arrows).

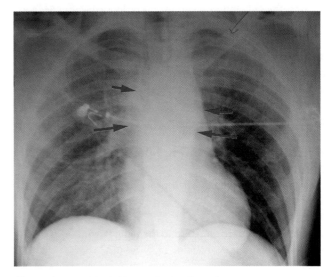

Abnormal paravertebral stripe on chest radiograph.

overaeration, bullous disease, or pneumothorax. Opaque hemithorax may result from collapse, consolidation, large masses, fibrosis, effusions, or haemothorax.

The lungs should be examined by looking at the three zones separately, comparing the right and left zones. Abnormal shadowing in the lungs can be classified broadly as linear, nodular, or having an air space pattern. Rarely, abnormal shadowing can be difficult to classify into one of these categories – under such circumstances, look at the peripheral aspect of the lungs. X rays cannot usually visualise structures <2 mm, so no vessels are seen in the peripheral 1-2 cm of the lungs, and this area should be examined for assessment of diffuse small opacities. High resolution computed tomography is often needed to provide better imaging in patients with diffuse lung disease, and computed tomography scanning is also helpful to characterise focal lesions.

Air space shadowing

This is also known as alveolar shadowing or consolidation. Air space shadowing is seen when the alveoli are filled with substances such as the ones listed below.

- Water: caused by cardiogenic or non-cardiogenic pulmonary oedema
- Pus: caused by infection, which could be bacterial, rarely viral, fungal, or protozoal
- Blood: caused by haemorrhage – for example, because of trauma, infarcts, vasculitis
- Eosinophils: caused by pulmonary eosinophilia – for example because of Loeffler's syndrome, drug reactions)
- Protein: caused by alveolar proteinosis
- Tumour: caused by alveolar cell carcinoma, lymphoma, or certain metastases
- Infiltration – non-malignant (for example, sarcoid, amyloid, or acute respiratory distress syndrome).

Lines

These are linear or curvilinear opacities within the lungs. Lines are characterised as follows.

- Septal lines are 1-2 mm thick and about 1-2 cm long (interstitial pulmonary oedema, lymphangitis carcinomatosa, or interstitial lung disease)
- *Atelectasis* – linear or band (subsegmental collapse)
- *Reticular* – lace-like pattern, usually longstanding (caused by fibrosing alveolitis, scleroderma, or drugs)
- *Honeycomb* – can be seen in chronic endstage lung disease
- *Rings* that are associated with tram lines indicate bronchiectasis
- *Rings* with no tram lines indicate cystic lung disease
- *Rings* that are pencil-thin resembling round cysts (pneumatocoeles)
- *Tubular* – vessels (serpigenous – arteriovenous malformations) or bronchi filled with pus (glove fingers).

Nodules

These are 1 mm-3 cm in diameter, whereas masses are >3 cm in diameter. The characteristics of nodules are:

- ≤1 mm: "micronodules," hyperdense as seen with alveolar microlithiasis

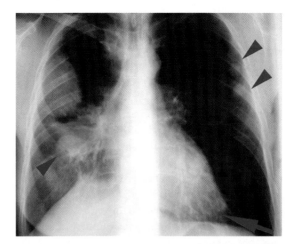

Left mastectomy (arrow) with transradiant left hemithorax, multiple metastasis (arrowheads), and a malignant right pleural effusion.

Lung pathology

- Air spaces – water, pus, blood, eosinophils, protein, tumour infiltration
- Nodules can be <2 mm, 2-3 mm, 3-5 mm, 5-30 mm (>30 mm is a mass)
- Lines can be dense linear (atelectasis), septal, rings and tram lines, cysts, or tubular or serpigenous

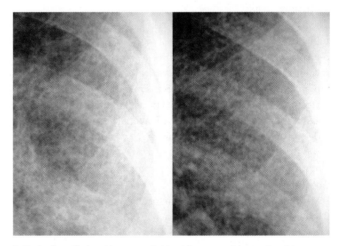

Reticular (lace-like) and honeycomb (rings) lines are evidence of endstage lung fibrosis (left). Miliary nodules (right).

- 2-3 mm: miliary – tuberculosis needs to be excluded first. These result from sarcoid, metastases, pneumoconiosis, atypical infections, drug reactions, and extrinsic allergic alveolitis
- 3 mm-3 cm: metastases or abscesses (rarely vasculitis or infarcts).

Masses

These are focal nodular lesions >3 cm in size. The causes of masses are:

- Primary bronchogenic carcinoma: most likely to occur in elderly people
- Abscess: most likely to occur in young, ill patients or immunosuppressed patients
- Haematoma is related to trauma with fractured ribs
- Arteriovenous malformations are rare with characteristic serpigenous vessels. They are usually solitary but, rarely, may be multiple
- Vasculitis: underlying diagnosis is usually known and is most likely rheumatoid arthritis or Wegener's granulomatosis
- Hamartomas have characteristic calcification (popcorn).

Trauma related conditions

Some of the common conditions related to trauma include flail segment, pneumothorax, haemothorax, lung contusion, pulmonary haematoma, pneumomediastinum, pericardial tamponade, traumatic aortic injury, and ruptured oesophagus.

Pneumothorax

The features of this condition are:

- Pleural edge visible
- No vessels beyond pleural edge
- Contralateral mediastinal shift and depression of ipsilateral hemidiaphragm suggests radiological tension
- On supine films there is increased lucency of hemithorax, depression and increased lucency of ipsilateral hemidiaphragm, and deep anterior costophrenic sulcus.

Pneumomediastinum

The features of this condition are:

- Streaks and bubbles of air within mediastinum
- Air outlining mediastinal vessels
- Air outlining the mediastinal pleura as linear shadow
- Air seen along superior aspect of diaphragm, giving appearance of continuous hemidiaphragm.

The causes of pneumomediastinum include alveolar rupture (asthma, ventilation, or trauma), tracheal injury (trauma), and oesophageal rupture (spontaneous or iatrogenic).

Traumatic aortic injury

The radiological features of this condition are divided into those that represent a medistinal haematoma and associated injuries.
Signs of mediastinal haematoma include:

- Mediastinal widening >8 cm at the level of aortic arch
- Mediastinum to chest ratio of >33%
- Deviation of the nasogastric tube and trachea to the right
- Depression of the left main bronchus
- Left apical pleural shadowing
- Loss of clarity or lobulated arch of the aorta.

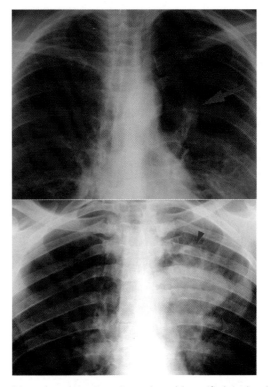

Primary bronchogenic carcinoma (arrow) (magnified view) and same view a year later (arrowheads).

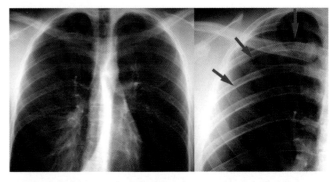

Pneumothorax (arrows) with magnified view (right).

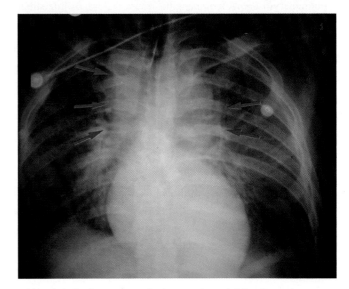

Widened mediastinum as a result of traumatic aortic injury (arrows).

Associated injuries include:

- Rib fractures
- Scapular, vertebral or sternum fractures
- Left haemothorax or effusion
- Left pneumothorax
- Lung contusion.

Some non-trauma related conditions

These include pleural effusions, pneumonia, heart failure, pulmonary emboli, and focal mass lesions.

Pleural effusion

The features of this condition are:

- Meniscus sign
- Thickened pleural space
- Obscuration of underlying lung
- Loculated pleural collections such as empyema will be seen as peripheral opacity with convex inner border and broad base
- On supine films, look for ill defined, hazy opacification with pulmonary vessels still visible, loss of clarity of ipsilateral hemidiaphragm, and apical pleural opacity.

Pulmonary air space opacification (consolidation)

The features of this condition are:

- 3-5 mm, ill defined nodular opacities
- Tendency of opacities to coalesce
- Loss of vascular markings
- Air bronchograms
- Obscuration of adjacent mediastinal borders and hemidiaphragm (silhouette)
- No volume loss.

The causes of consolidation include infection, pulmonary oedema, haemorrhage, pulmonary infarction, tumours, eosinophilic lung disease, and other causes, such as sarcoidosis and alveolar proteinosis.

Heart failure (pulmonary oedema)

The features of this condition are:

- Cardiac enlargement
- Basal vasoconstriction
- Upper lobe blood diversion
- Loss of clarity of pulmonary vessels (perivascular haziness)
- Thickening of bronchi (peribronchical cuffing)
- Kerley A lines: thin linear opacities in the mid and upper zones radiating out from the hila
- Kerley B lines: linear opacities 1-2 cm long, 1-2 mm thick, perpendicular to pleural surface caused by interstitial fluid
- Pleural effusions
- Perihilar consolidation.

The causes of this condition include cardiac failure, fluid overload, aspiration, re-expansion after rapid thoracocentesis, near drowning, inhalation of noxious gases, adult respiratory distress syndrome, raised intracranial pressure (neurogenic).

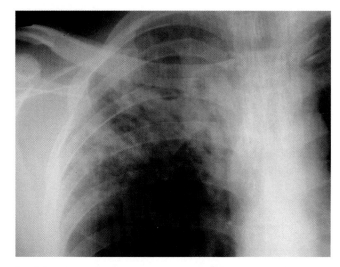

Focal air space opacity.

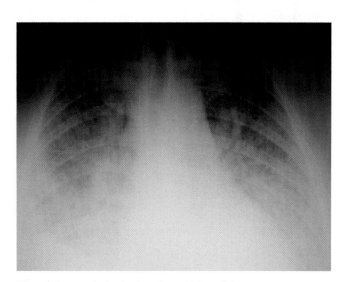

Bilateral air space shadowing in patient with heart failure.

Pulmonary collapse

The features of this condition are:

· Increased opacification of involved lobe or lung
· Volume loss that may manifest as tracheal or hilar shift, elevation of the hemidiaphragm, and shift of the mediastinum or fissures.
· Compensatory hyperinflation of other lobes or lung
· Loss of volume of the involved lobe, which may manifest as crowding of ribs, mediastinal shift, or displacement of the hila and fissures.

The causes of this condition include primary bronchogenic carcinoma, other endobronchial tumours (for example, carcinoid tumours), foreign bodies, mucus plugging, compression of airways by extrinsic mass, secondary to pleural effusion or pneumothorax.

Pulmonary masses

The features of this condition are:

· Multiple lesions – suggests metastases (rarely abscesses)
· Calcification – makes bronchial carcinoma unlikely
· Irregular or spiculated edge suggests bronchogenic carcinoma
· Cavitation suggests lung abscess and carcinoma
· Invasion of chest wall indicates bronchogenic carcinoma
· Rapid growth of mass suggests an abscess
· Growth over months to two years indicates carcinoma or metastases
· Lack of growth of mass over two years suggests benign lesion
· Serpigenous vessel indicates arteriovenous malformations
· Mass containing fat density or fat or popcorn calcification suggests a hamartoma.

The causes of this condition include bronchial carcinoma, metastatic deposit, other bronchial neoplasms (for example, carcinoid neoplasm), benign tumours (for example, hamartoma), tuberculoma, lung abscess, vasculitis (Wegener's granulomatosis), rheumatoid arthritis.

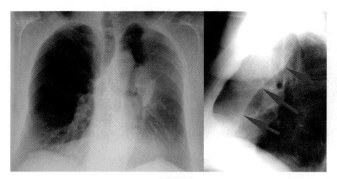

Frontal (left) and lateral (right) chest radiographs showing collapse of left upper lobe. There is diffuse opacification of the left hemithorax, loss of outline of the left heart border, and anteriror displacement of the oblique fissure (arrows).

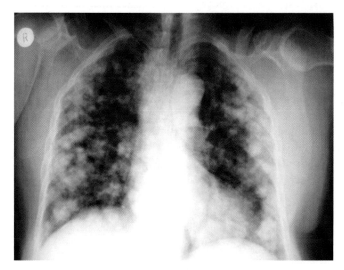

Lung metastases – multiple large and small lesions.

CHAPTER 11

Abdomen

Niall Power, Tim Fotheringham, Otto Chan

Despite the advent of technologies such as ultrasonography, computed tomography, and magnetic resonance imaging (MRI), the abdominal radiograph remains an important investigation for abdominal symptoms and is often the only study required. The abdominal radiograph lacks the symmetry of the chest and has a wide range of normal appearances. Thus, a systematic approach to assessment is essential. This chapter covers this approach and summarises common acute emergency conditions. The trend nowadays, however, is to do an abdominal radiograph and then, if clinically indicated, to go straight to computed tomography (or ultrasonography). Magnetic resonance imaging has no important role in the initial management of abdominal emergencies.

Anatomy

Normal appearances of abdominal radiographs vary, but the boxes below show some useful general points to remember when assessing the radiographs.

Positions of solid organs

Organ	Position	Appearance on radiograph
Liver	Right upper quadrant	Subhepatic edge visible, rarely extends to iliac crest
Spleen	Left upper quadrant	Rarely seen below twelfth rib
Kidneys	Flanks	Readily visible, outlined by fat and psoas (L1-4), left higher
Pancreas	Central	Not visible and retroperitoneal
Uterus	Pelvis	Usually outlined by fat above bladder

Indications for abdominal radiography

- Abdominal pain
- Suspected small bowel obstruction
- Suspected large bowel obstruction
- Palpable mass
- Renal or ureteric colic

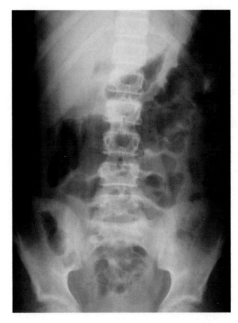

Anteroposterior abdominal radiograph.

Positions of hollow organs

Organ	Position	Appearance on radiograph
Stomach	Upper, central	Lies transverse across upper abdomen
Small bowel	Mid central	<3 cm wide, not usually visible
Large bowel	Peripheral	Contains air and faeces, outlined by properitoneal fat
Bladder	Lower central	Outlined by perivesical fat

The structures in the abdomen are visible mainly because bowel gas and fat planes separate them. The abdomen is usually divided into the peritoneal cavity, the pelvic cavity, and the retroperitoneal space. These cavities cannot be differentiated on an abdominal radiograph, although pathology can be identified. To localise the abnormalities, computed tomography is generally required, although ultrasonography can be helpful.

ABCs systematic assessment

- Adequacy
- Air
- Bowel
- Calcification
- Densities
- Edges
- Fat planes
- Skeleton, solid organs

Adequacy

The standard radiograph is an anteroposterior view taken with the patient supine. Erect abdominal radiographs used to be performed routinely, but they are now largely obsolete. If the plain supine abdominal radiograph is featureless, however, an erect abdominal radiograph may be helpful in showing fluid levels.

The erect chest radiograph is mandatory if the patient's complaint is abdominal pain, because it is an extremely useful view to find free intraperitoneal air (pneumoperitoneum). Small amounts of free air can be seen under the hemidiaphragm if enough time (at least 10 minutes) is allowed for the free air to rise. If the patient is too ill to stand up, a left lateral decubitus view (left side down) can be taken to look for free air. The erect chest radiograph may sometimes show pathology in the chest simulating an acute abdomen, such as pneumonia or aortic dissection.

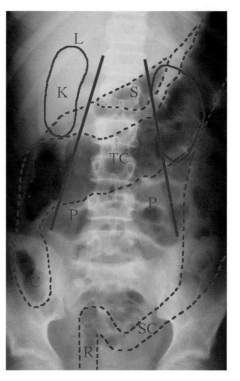

Hollow organs, solid organs, and fat planes – C=caecum, K=kidney, L=liver, LB=large bowel, S=stomach, SB=small bowel, SC=sigmoid colon, and R=rectum.

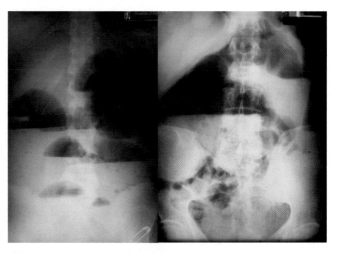

Erect abdominal radiographs showing dilated small bowel (left) and dilated large bowel (right).

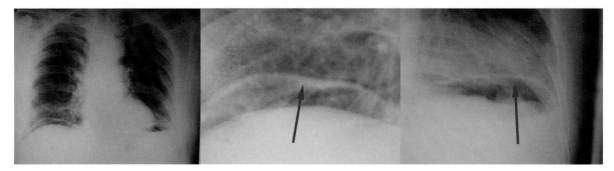

Erect chest radiographs with free air (arrows) under both diaphragms (left) and magnified views of hemidiaphragms (middle and right).

A rapid initial assessment of the adequacy of the radiograph should be made. A technically adequate film should include the pubic symphyses and show the hernial orifices and the properitoneal fat planes. These fat planes are thin layers of fat between the parietal peritoneum and the lateral wall muscles. An additional view of the upper abdomen may be necessary in tall patients. The following should then be assessed:

- **A**ir – exclude free intraperitoneal and retroperitoneal air
- **B**owel – gas pattern, size, and distribution. Exclude small bowel and large bowel obstruction
- **C**alcifications – check renal tract, vascular, and other structures
- **D**ensities – look for tablets and foreign bodies
- **E**dges – check hernial orifices
- **F**at planes – check psoas, properitoneal, and perivesical fat planes
- **S**keleton – look at the bones for fractures.
- **S**olid organs – look for liver, spleen, and kidneys.

Air

Free intraperitoneal air rises to the front of the abdomen on a supine abdominal radiograph. This free air can be hard to detect, so an erect chest radiograph is essential if perforation is suspected. Look for extraluminal air.

Bowel

Gas pattern

When the patient is supine, bowel gas rises to the parts of the gastrointestinal tract that are most anterior. These parts include the stomach, transverse colon, and sigmoid colon. The stomach is located above the transverse colon and has band-like rugal folds across it. The small bowel can be differentiated from the large bowel by the following features:

- Position: the small bowel lies in the centre of the abdomen; the large bowel lies peripherally.
- Size: the small bowel is smaller than the large bowel in calibre. The jejunum should measure <3.5 cm, the ileum <3 cm, and the distal ileum <2.5 cm. The large bowel has no definite measurement, but if the caecum dilates to more than 9 cm, it infers impending perforation if an obstruction is present. In the presence of colitis, any part of the colon that measures more than 5.5 cm indicates a megacolon, but the normal colon can easily be larger than this.
- Pattern: the dilated jejunum and proximal ileum have characteristic thin folds (valvulae conniventes) that run across the whole bowel. These folds are closer together than the thicker folds (haustrae) of the large bowel. The haustrae do not run across the whole dilated large bowel. The distal ileum and sigmoid colon are relatively featureless.
- Content: the small bowel contains fluid and air, whereas the colon contains faeces, which has a characteristic appearance.

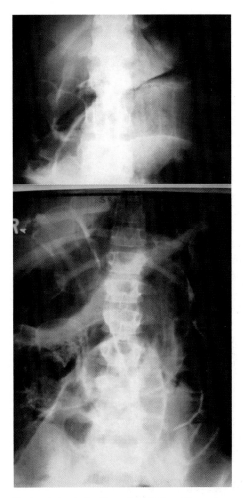

Supine abdominal radiographs with free air.

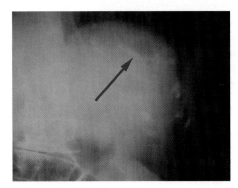

Costal cartilage.

Calcification

Many normal and abnormal structures in the abdomen can calcify. These include:

- Costal cartilage can sometimes be seen in the upper abdomen as an incidental finding.
- Phleboliths are small calcified veins in the pelvis. They can be confused with ureteric stones.
- Coarse, nodular calcification in mesenteric lymph nodes is an incidental finding lying between the left L2 transverse process and the lower right sacroiliac joint.
- Vascular calcification: this type of calcification is curvilinear and often seen in the aorta.
- More than 90% of renal and ureteric calculi are visible on a radiograph.
- Only 10-15% of gallstones are radio-opaque. Rarely, the gallbladder wall can calcify (porcelain gall bladder).
- Punctate fine stippled nodular calcification in the pancreas indicates chronic pancreatitis.
- Calcification in the spleen is usually caused by previous trauma or infections such as granulomatous or parasitic.
- Appendicoliths are important to detect. They are usually seen in the right iliac fossa, and, in the correct clinical context, they are evidence of acute appendicitis. Appendicoliths often imply a complicated appendicitis – for example, a mass or abscess. Even in the absence of symptoms, patients with an appendicolith should be referred to the surgeon for an appendicectomy.
- Tuberculosis and schistosomiasis infections can cause calcification of the bladder wall.

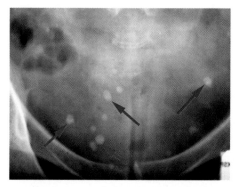

Phleboliths.

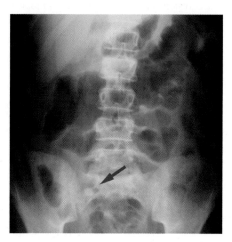

Appendicolith.

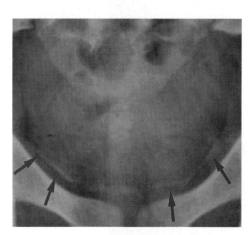

Calcification of the bladder wall.

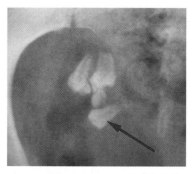

Dermoid with teeth.

- Teeth can sometimes be seen in dermoid cysts, and rarely ovarian tumours can calcify.
- Calcification of the seminal vesicles is often seen in patients with diabetes or renal failure.
- Uterus: it is common for fibroids to calcify as large masses in the lower pelvis.

Densities

These include foreign bodies, tablets, and tampons. Foreign bodies of any type can be ingested or inserted via any orifice. Tablets often contain calcium. Tampons can be seen as tubular structures filled with air in the lower pelvis.

Edges

In particular, look at the hernial orifices for a bowel in hernia (this is a common cause of small bowel obstruction). Central lines are sometimes inserted via the groin.

Fat planes

Identification of normal fat planes is important because their distortion or displacement can indicate pathology. Visible fat planes include:

- Psoas: these are seen easily in most abdominal radiographs. Any asymmetry or displacement is an important finding and usually indicates an abnormality in the retroperitoneum or the adjacent spine. The right psoas may not be visible in 20% of abdominal radiographs.
- Perirenal fat plane: kidneys are obvious on radiographs, and any enlargement, atrophy, or displacement should be visible.

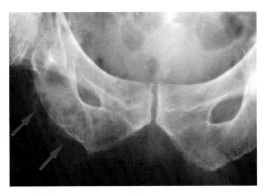

Small bowel in hernia.

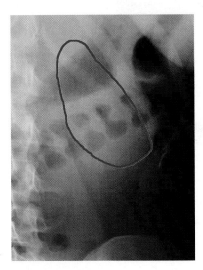

Perirenal fat plane.

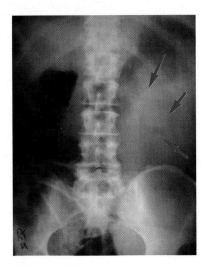

Displaced psoas.

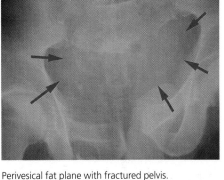

Perivesical fat plane with fractured pelvis.

- Displacement of the perivesical fat plane indicates a pelvic haematoma, and (in the trauma setting) a probable fracture.
- Properitoneal fat planes lie outside the parietal peritoneum and, on a radiograph, outline the ascending and descending colon.
- Other solid organs: most solid organs can be seen on a radiograph if a fat plane separates an organ from the adjacent structures. For example, the liver, spleen, and uterus (but not the pancreas) are surrounded by fat planes.

Skeleton

After trauma, fractures are important to detect because they indicate the possibility of a solid or hollow organ injury. About 30% of patients with a fracture of the lower three ribs have an intra-abdominal injury that can be detected with computed tomography. Conversely, one third of patients with liver and spleen injuries that have been detected with computed tomography have a rib fracture.

In trauma patients abdominal radiographs are not indicated routinely. Only a pelvic radiograph is necessary unless a patient has a penetrating injury. Knives should be left in the wound and imaged. In patients with gunshot wounds, the entry and exit sites of the bullets should be marked with paper clips.

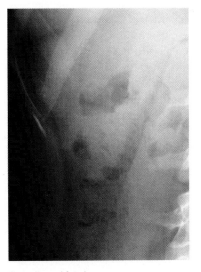

Properitoneal fat plane.

Common abdominal emergencies

Dilated small bowel

The most common causes of dilated small bowel loops are mechanical obstruction and paralytic ileus. Mechanical obstruction of the small bowel may be caused by:

- Adhesions (75% of all causes)
- Strangulated hernias
- Abdominal masses
- Small bowel volvulus and intussusception
- Gallstone ileus and inflammatory processes, such as Crohn's disease and appendix abscesses.

The cardinal features of small bowel obstruction are dilated loops of small bowel (usually >3 cm in diameter) containing variable amounts of air and fluid, with collapse of the large bowel. Air-fluid levels >2.5 cm in length also indicate an obstruction. As the air is resorbed with increasing duration of obstruction, small amounts of residual air become trapped between valvulae conniventes and look like "a string of beads." Small bowel obstruction can be difficult to differentiate from paralytic ileus. In the latter, the large bowel is also often dilated, and the string of beads sign is rarely seen. Computed tomography should be done in all patients with suspected small bowel obstruction.

Dilated large bowel

In patients with paralytic ileus, the large bowel can be dilated. Pseudo-obstruction is a form of ileus and is characterised by dilatation of the colon without an obstructing lesion. Common causes of large bowel obstruction include carcinoma, volvulus, and inflammatory processes (for example, diverticular disease).

Patients with these conditions are at high risk of perforation of the large bowel, especially if the diameter of the caecum exceeds 9 cm. A competent ileo-caecal valve will prevent decompression of the dilated caecum into the distal ileum and increase the risk of perforation. Volvulus is the twisting of a bowel loop, and it affects loops with redundant and long mesentery. The most common sites in which volvulus may occur are the caecum and sigmoid colon, and it causes a closed loop obstruction. The caecum can rotate anywhere with associated small bowel obstruction. The redundant loop of sigmoid classically rotates towards the left upper quadrant to give an inverted U appearance, devoid of haustra, with a characteristic central stripe that results from the adjacent bowel walls. Proximal large bowel obstruction is often seen. Dilated large bowel can also be seen in acute colitis, usually ulcerative colitis, where it is associated with wall thickening and mucosal oedema and produces an appearance of "thumbprinting." This is known as toxic megacolon, and perforation of the large bowel is often imminent.

If large bowel obstruction is suspected, computed tomography is the investigation of choice after the abdominal radiograph. If pseudo-obstruction or paralytic ileus are suspected, however, a follow-up film or limited single contrast enema is a good alternative.

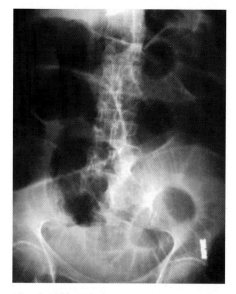

Dilated small bowel.

Causes of small bowel dilatation

- Small bowel obstruction
  Adhesions (commonest cause)
  Strangulated hernias
  Gallstone ileus (occurs in 25% of elderly patients)
  Tumours
  Intussusception
  Crohn's disease
  Volvulus
- Paralytic ileus
- Mesenteric infarction
- Meteorrhistic bowel (often seen in children who cry and swallow air)

Causes of large bowel dilatation

- Large bowel obstruction
  Carcinoma
  Diverticular disease
  Adhesions
  Volvulus (usually sigmoid and rarely caecum)
  Radiotherapy
- Paralytic ileus
- Pseudo-obstruction
- Meteorrhistic bowel
- Toxic megacolon

Extraluminal air

Air outside the lumen of the bowel has an array of causes of varying clinical significance. These include:

Free intraperitoneal air – Implies a perforation, usually of a peptic ulcer or diverticulitis, unless the patient has recently undergone laparotomy. Free air can be difficult to see on a supine radiograph and if you are concerned, an erect chest radiograph should be obtained.

Air may be seen on the supine film in the hepatorenal recess (Morrison's pouch) or between bowel loops. Rigler's sign visualises both sides of the bowel wall caused by the presence of air on either side of it (normally fat abuts the outside of the wall and the wall cannot be distinguished).

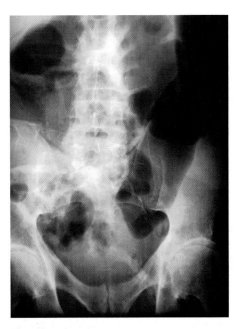

Dilated large bowel.

Signs of free intraperitoneal air on supine abdominal radiographs

- Rigler's sign – both sides of the bowel wall can be seen
- Unicupola sign – air in the central leaf of the diaphragm
- Subhepatic air – free air under the inferior margin of the liver
- Football sign – air lies under the anterior abdominal wall
- Falciform ligament – air outlines the falciform ligament over the liver

---

Air in the bowel wall – May reflect the benign condition known as pneumatosis cystoides intestinalis or pneumatosis cystoides coli if the air is in a spherical or oval configuration; but linear streaks of intramural air are important as they usually indicate infarction of the bowel wall, which may be a sequela of severe inflammation or ischaemia. Ischaemic colitis affects elderly patients, usually in the region of the splenic flexure, and it manifests as thickening of the bowel wall and thumbprinting before the development of pneumatosis.

Other causes – Gas in the portal venous system should be differentiated from air in the biliary system (aerobilia) because of its peripheral location in the liver. This is a sinister sign in the adult patient that indicates transmural bowel infarction with tracking of air into the mesenteric veins.

Aerobilia and air in the gallbladder can be caused by placement of a biliary stent or erosion of a gallstone through the gallbladder wall into the small bowel. This may cause small bowel obstruction – a condition known as gallstone ileus.

Air may also be seen in an abscess, where it may have a mottled appearance or produce an abnormal air-fluid level. An abscess may have mass effect and displace adjacent structures. It should be suspected from the clinical history and presentation. Computed tomography or ultrasonography are the investigations of choice if an abscess is suspected.

Gastrointestinal emergencies

Gallstone ileus

Gallstone ileus is a rare cause of small bowel obstruction, except in the elderly population (occurs in up to 25% of the elderly population). Typically the gallbladder has become chronically inflamed and erodes into the small bowel, usually the duodenum. The stone passes into the small bowel, and then obstructs just proximal to the

---

Causes of extraluminal air

Free intraperitoneal air (pneumoperitoneum)
- Perforated viscus duodenal ulcer or diverticulitis
- Postobstruction (large bowel and small bowel)
- Mesenteric ischaemia
- Ischaemic colitis
- Iatrogenic (laparoscopy, hysterosalpingography, or percutaneous transhepatic cholangiography)
- Pneumatosis coli (asymptomatic)

Bowel (subserosal)
- Pneumatosis coli
- Pneumatosis intestinalis

Bowel (intramural)
- Necrotising enterocolitis
- Ischaemic colitis

Aerobilia
- Emphysematous cholecystitis
- After endoscopic retrograde cholangiopancreatography or sphincterotomy
- Gallstone ileus

Renal tract
- Emphysematous pyelonephritis or cystitis

Genitourinary tract (women)
- Tampons
- Douching
- Hysterosalpingograms

ileo-caecal valve. The hallmarks are dilated small bowel, air in the biliary tree, and (rarely) the stone is radio-opaque.

Mesenteric infarction

This causes severe abdominal pain in elderly patients with arrhythmias, or young patients who have embolic episodes from a tumour (atrial myxoma), vasculitis, or bacterial endocarditis. Usually, only dilated loops of the small bowel are seen initially, but later, air in the bowel wall and portal vein gas may be seen.

Contrast-enhanced computed tomography, computed tomography angiography or mesenteric angiography are necessary to make the diagnosis.

Pseudo-obstruction

Mimics large bowel obstruction, but no cause is found. It is often seen in elderly patients. It is a diagnosis of exclusion with computed tomography, single contrast enema, or colonoscopy.

Paralytic ileus

As above, except patients have no bowel sounds, and sometimes they have biochemical abnormalities. It occurs in particular after surgery.

Gastric volvulus

The stomach rotates around itself and can end up in any part of the abdomen. The hallmarks are usually a single distended viscus and an absent normal stomach. Diagnosis is generally made with an abdominal radiograph and repeat radiograph after a nasogastric tube insertion.

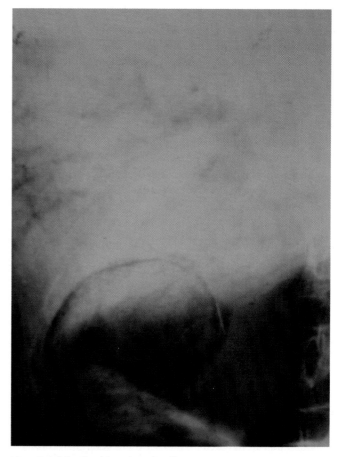

Mesenteric infarction (air on bowel wall).

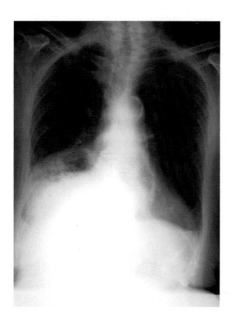

Gastric volvulus.

Caecal volvulus

The caecum is mobile and rotates with its mesentery. The hallmarks are a distended air-filled viscus and dilated small bowel and an absent normal caecum. Diagnosis is made using an abdominal

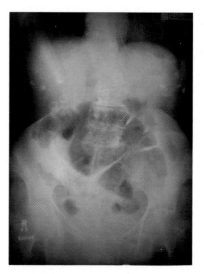

Caecal volvulus.

radiograph and, if necessary, a single contrast enema (or computed tomography).

Sigmoid volvulus

The sigmoid colon is mobile and elongated in elderly patients and intermittently rotates on itself and the mesentery pedicle.

The abdominal radiograph appearances are classic, with a grossly dilated double loop of large bowel arising from the left side of the pelvis extending onto the left upper abdomen, the apex lies above T10 and the liver (liver overlap sign) and descending colon (bowel overlap sign) can be seen through these dilated loops.

Diagnosis is made with the abdominal radiograph, but a single contrast enema can be done to confirm the diagnosis (bird of prey sign) if necessary.

Ischaemic colitis

Usually affects the splenic and descending colon and leads to a functional obstruction with associated thumbprinting of the colon. In advanced cases, there may be bowel wall air, portal vein gas and a pneumoperitoneum. An abdominal radiograph is helpful.

Inflammatory colitis

Faeces is absent in the affected colon with abnormal mucosa (pseudopolyps), thumbprints, and associated megacolon visible on the plain abdominal radiograph. Colonoscopy and follow-up abdominal radiographs are indicated.

Acute appendicitis

If an abdominal radiograph is done, there is sometimes a dilated small bowel loop (sentinel loop) overlying the inflamed appendix. It is not routinely indicated, but atypical presentations may also show an appendicolith or a mass on an abdominal radiograph. Computed tomography is the investigation of choice if the diagnosis is in doubt, compression ultrasonography in thin adults, pregnant women, and children is an alternative.

Others

Trauma

An abdominal radiograph is not indicated. A pelvic radiograph and focussed abdominal sonography for trauma (FAST) should be done as part of the primary survey. In major trauma computed tomography should be performed in most patients (see chapter 17).

Biliary colic and acute cholecystitis

As above, an abdominal radiograph is not indicated. Ultrasonography is the investigation of choice or isotope cholescintigraphy in acute cholecystitis.

Acute pancreatitis

An abdominal radiograph is not indicated. Ultrasonography should be done to look for gallstones and to exclude a dilated biliary system, but it is not performed to look at the pancreas.

If an abdominal radiograph is done, there is sometimes a dilated small bowel loop (sentinel loop) overlying the inflamed pancreas or calcification indicating underlying chronic pancreatitis.

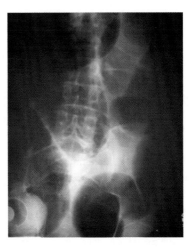

Sigmoid volvulus.

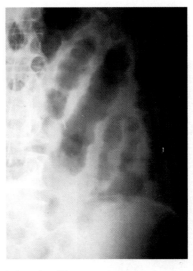

Ischaemic colitis.

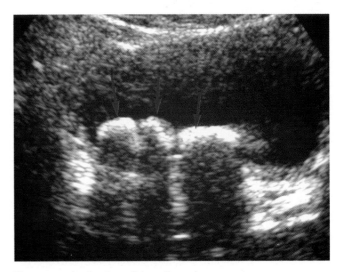

Ultrasonography showing gallstones (arrows).

Leaking abdominal aortic aneurysm

The curvilinear calcification of the aneurysm is usually visible, but there are many other features to suggest that there is a leak – a soft tissue mass around the calcified wall (haematoma), loss of the psoas (left in particular), displaced left kidney superiorly and outwards, and displacement of bowel loops to the periphery (by the haematoma).

Renal or ureteric colic

An abdominal radiograph is not indicated. Preferably, computed tomography of the kidneys, ureters, and bladder (CT KUB) or an emergency (limited) intravenous urography should be done. The CT KUB is a limited computed tomogram with no contrast, a low dose, and can detect up to 15% of additional abnormalities to intravenous urography.

Masses

Initially ultrasonography is performed to identify the origin of the mass. All females of child bearing age should be considered pregnant until proven otherwise. Ultrasonography scan can detect a 3-4 week old pregnancy and a heart beat can be seen at five weeks.

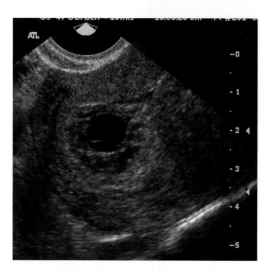

Ultrasonography at six weeks' gestation.

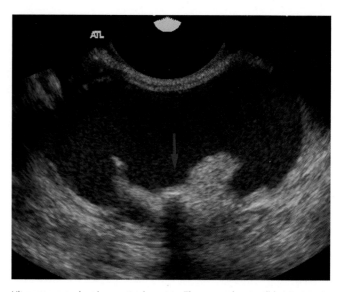

Ultrasonogram showing an ovarian mass. The arrow shows solid component.

ABCs systematic assessment

Air
- Exclude free intraperitoneal or abnormal sited air

Bowel gas
- Check size, distribution, and pattern

Calcification
- Check for normal and abnormal calcification

Densities
- Check for inserted or ingested foreign bodies

Edges
- Check the hernial orifices
- Check for lung base pathology such as metastases or collapsed lung

Fat planes
- Check symmetry of psoas shadows
- Check presence of perivesical fat plane
- Check that properitoneal fat planes are present

Soft tissues
- Check for enlarged or absent organs. Confirm with ultrasonography

Skeleton
- In trauma, check that there are no obvious fractures
- If malignancy is suspected, exclude skeletal involvement

CHAPTER 12

Head

Amrish Mehta, Otto Chan

Most patients that require head imaging present to the emergency department after trauma, suspected stroke, transient ischaemic attack, suspected subarachnoid haemorrhage, or meningitis. Computed tomography (CT) is the mainstay of cranial imaging in the acute or emergency clinical setting. Other than in stroke, magnetic resonance imaging has no significant role in the initial management of patients with these conditions.

CT technique

When CT is being carried out, the patient is moved through the scanner, usually supine, and images are obtained with a rotating x ray tube and detectors. The latest CT scanners have 64 detectors and can rotate 360° in 0.4 seconds, generating 160 images per second or 9600 images per minute. Nevertheless, axial images of the head are usually acquired "sequentially" with one rotation of the detector per slice.

Initially, a scout image (scanogram) is obtained. The patient then has axial images taken through the head from the foramen magnum to the vertex. In the emergency setting, images are initially acquired without intravenous contrast enhancement (non-enhanced CT). The scans are then reviewed and, if necessary, intravenous contrast (iodine based) is administered (contrast enhanced CT). Non-enhanced CT with or without subsequent intravenous contrast administration is indicated in a variety of clinical scenarios.

The key to the diagnosis of an intracranial abnormality is knowledge of basic anatomy of the head and axial CT anatomy of the head.

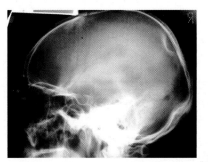
Lateral skull radiograph showing focal depressed fracture of the parietal bone.

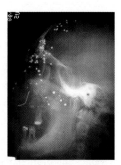
Lateral skull radiograph showing lead gunshot injury with multiple foci of high density projected over the face.

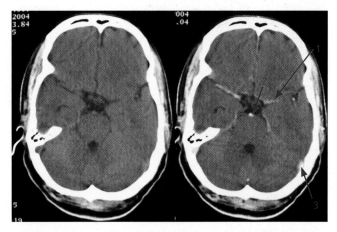
Computed tomogram of the head before (left) and after (right) intravenous contrast administration. On this slice, the middle cerebral arteries (1) basilar artery (2) and lateral venous sinuses (3) are shown as high density structures after contrast as is the free edge of the tentorium.

Indications for CT of the head

Non-enhanced CT	Non-enhanced CT with or without contrast enhanced CT
• Trauma (including non-accidental injury) • Subarachnoid haemorrhage • Intracranial haemorrhage • Stroke • Hypoxia • Anoxia	• Meningitis • Raised intracranial pressure • Obstructive hydrocephalus • After neurosurgery

Non-enhanced CT and contrast enhanced CT	Contrast enhanced CT or magnetic resonance imaging
• Encephalitis (acute confusion) • Subdural empyema • Venous sinus thrombosis • Known primary malignancy • HIV infection • Focal mass legion	• Focal lesion • Subdural empyema • Encephalitis • Venous sinus thrombosis • HIV infection

ABCDEF systematic assessment – primary assessment of cranial CT

- **A**irspaces
- **B**ones and **b**rain parenchyma
- **C**erebrospinal fluid spaces
- **D**ural spaces
- **E**yes
- **F**ace, **f**oreign bodies

Several integral steps aid accurate interpretation of cranial CT imaging. The first step is the development of a safe and reproducible system of initial assessment. The ABC assessment is systematic, simple, and easy to remember. It is important to review key areas analogous to a secondary survey. Understanding anatomy and determining whether a lesion is intrinsic (in brain parenchyma) or extra-axial (in the dural or cerebrospinal fluid spaces) is crucial.

An appreciation of the range of normal appearances, typical imaging artefacts (such as "beam hardening" in the posterior fossa and temporal lobes and "partial voluming" in the inferior frontal lobes and next to the petrous ridge), and patterns of abnormalities is essential. Although the method presented here was developed for interpreting cranial CT in the trauma setting, it can be used in other situations.

Airspaces

Check:
- Sphenoid sinus: a fluid level may indicate a base of skull fracture.
- Other paranasal sinuses: opacification of the air sinuses may be due to sinusitis and may be the cause of a subdural empyema (infected subdural fluid collection). Maxillary antrum and ethmoid air cell opacification is often seen with facial fractures.
- Mastoid air cells and petrous bones: opacification here is a strong indicator of a petrous bone fracture in trauma. Opacification and bone erosion may represent a skull base tumour, such as a chondrosarcoma or metastasis, or an infective process such as petrous apicitis.

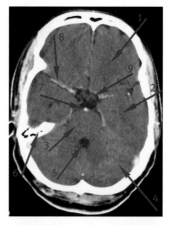

Contrast enhanced computed tomogram of head (1=frontal lobes, 2=temporal lobes, 3=pons, 4=cerebellar hemisphere, 5=fourth ventricle, 6=right petrous bone, 7=basilar artery, 8=right middle cerebral artery, 9=optic chiasm).

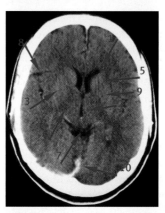

Axial CT scan of head. (1=frontal horn of lateral ventricle, 2=third ventricle, 3=right putamen, 4=head of right caudate nucleus, 5=anterior limb of left internal capsule, 6=posterior limb of right internal capsule, 7=quadrageminal cistern, 8=right sylvian fissure, 9=left globus pallidus, 10 torcula (confluence of venous sinuses).

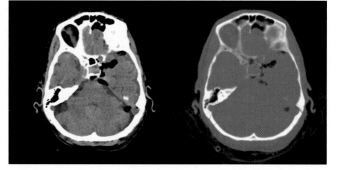

Pneumocephalus. Pockets of very low density (jet black) in the extra-axial spaces on both the soft tissue (left) and bone window (right) settings.

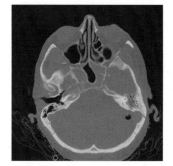

Longitudinal fracture of the left petrous temporal bone with opacification of the mastoid air cells and middle ear cleft, and pneumocephalus.

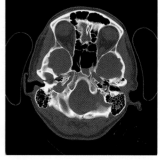

Fracture of the left lateral wall of the sphenoid sinus with a fluid level within the sinus.

- Pneumocephalus: air in the skull usually indicates previous surgical intervention (commonly craniotomy, insertion of a ventricular drain or intracranial pressure monitoring device) or a fracture of a wall of an airspace (for example, sinus or aerated petrous bone).

Bones

It is important to examine the bones of a cranial CT study only on the bone window setting (window width 500, window level 1500), and ideally on images that have been reconstructed using a bone algorithm.

Check for:

- Scalp soft tissue swelling. This is often a marker for acute injury.
- Depressed or embedded bone fragments. These may need neurosurgical intervention, particularly if the degree of depression is >1 cm.
- Fractures or erosions at the skull base. Assess the foramina, carotid canals and petrous bones and clivus. The bony margins of the pituitary fossa may be eroded and remodelled by a large pituitary mass.
- Multiple fractures or abnormalities.
- Generalised skull vault thickening – for example, this may be seen in Paget's disease, diffuse metastatic disease (especially prostate carcinoma), sickle cell disease, anticonvulsant therapy, or long term ventricular shunting.
- Sclerotic or lucent bone lesions. The important diagnoses here are metastatic lesions and multiple myeloma.

When assessing the bones for fractures, do not mistake them for sutures. Sutures are typically symmetrical, less straight and have corticated edges.

Brain parenchyma

Examination of the brain parenchyma on every axial image for evidence of low density or high density lesions or for mass effect is necessary. In the trauma setting, low density lesions such as non-haemorrhagic confusions or "shear" injuries are typical. The latter include diffuse axonal injury which often occurs at the grey-white matter junction in the frontal and temporal lobes and in the corpus callosum, usually posteriorly. In non-trauma cases, low density lesions may involve grey and white matter (such as infarcts, encephalitis, and low grade gliomas) or white matter only. Demyelination and small vessel ischaemic disease in hypertension are common causes of white matter low density lesions. Vasogenic oedema is an area of low density around an abscess or tumour which has finger-like projections in the white matter. Diffuse low attenuation change with reduced grey-white matter differentiation and associated generalised cerebral swelling usually indicates hypoxic brain injury – for example, after prolonged cardiac arrest.

Further focal low attenuation may be related to cystic lesions, for example, cystic tumours, such as pilocytic astrocytoma, or to areas of necrosis in more aggressive tumours such as glioblastoma multiforme. Similarly, an abscess has a low density core with a thin enhancing wall.

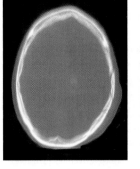

Computed tomogram showing comminuted fracture of the left parietal bone.

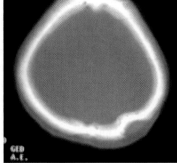

Computed tomogram of the patient in the figure at the top of the chapter, showing depressed fracture of the left parietal bone.

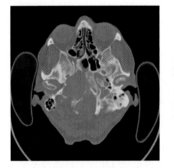

Metastasis – large expansile lytic lesion of the right side of the skull base.

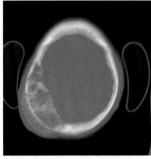

Haemangioma in the vault of the skull – large expansile lucent lesion of the right parietal bone with coarsened trabecular pattern and almost a "hair on end" appearance, which is typical.

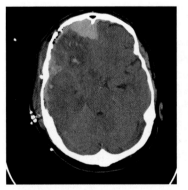

Mixed density elements in the right frontal and temporal lobes following trauma. The low density areas are non-haemorrhagic contusions. Note the right frontal extra-axial haematoma underlying the right frontal fracture.

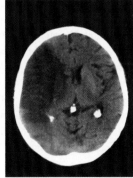

Subacute right middle cerebral artery territory infarct with low attenuation involving grey and white matter and associated with local mass effect.

High density lesions

High density lesions usually represent acute haemorrhage. Certainly from day 1 to day 7, a haemorrhage will be of high attenuation. In the acute setting, there may be associated surrounding low density – for example, non-haemorrhagic contusion, venous infarct, or haemorrhagic tumour. The density of the haemorrhage progressively reduces with time such that it may not be conspicuous at three to four weeks. In cases of ongoing parenchymal bleeding or in the presence of a coagulopathy, hyperacute haemorrhage can be of low density and may form fluid levels and "swirls." An acute haemorrhage may be less dense than expected in the context of anaemia. Alternatively, very high density areas may reflect calcification, possibly from congenital infection, or they could be related to a tumour. Lesions with high cellular density (for example, lymphoma) are often mildly hyperdense, and they usually have mass effect.

Mass effect

Deciding if a lesion has mass effect or if there is evidence of mass effect (without necessarily appreciating the causative lesion) is crucial. If a lesion has mass effect it causes distortion of adjacent structures, initially locally, but when more severe there is a more widespread effect. Common signs of mass effect are:

- Gyral expansion
- Cerebrospinal fluid space effacement (local or generalised effect on sulci, basal cistern and ventricles)
- Subfalcine herniation
- Crowding of the foramen magnum
- Temporal uncal herniation, which may result in a posterior cerebral artery infarct.

Cerebrospinal fluid spaces

The ventricles, basal cisterns, and sulci contain cerebrospinal fluid. All components should be assessed for signs of acute haemorrhage (high density) or mass effect. Acute haemorrhage in the basal cisterns, sulci with or without ventricles is a subarachnoid haemorrhage, the most common causes of which are trauma and cerebral aneurysm rupture. Take care to look in the dependent locations, particularly the occipital horns of the lateral ventricles and the interpeduncular fossa. Haemorrhage in the sulci results in high density linear lesions between the cortical gyri. Mass effect on the cerebrospinal fluid spaces usually results in the loss of symmetry – for example, of the ventricular system or sulci. The spaces are relatively small in normal young patients, so changes may be subtle.

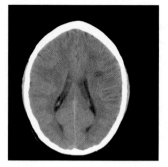

Small ovoid areas of low attenuation in the deep cerebral white matter. Not a specific appearance on computed tomogram, but suggests demyelination. Confirmed with magnetic resonance imaging.

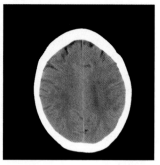

Small vessel ischaemia – several small areas of low attenuation in the deep and subcortical white matter of both cerebral hemispheres in an elderly patient with multiple vascular risk factors.

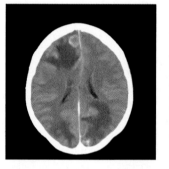

Vasogenic oedema – finger-like areas of low attenuation involving white matter is typical of this process. There are peripherally enhancing metastases that cause the oedematous reaction.

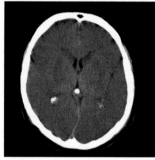

Severe hypoxic brain injury. Symmetric low attenuation involving the basal ganglia. It is associated with cerebral swelling, and loss of the differentiation of grey and white matter in keeping with generalised cerebral oedema.

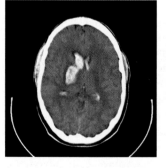

Acute parenchymal haemorrhage. High density acute haematoma in the right basal ganglia but with intraventricular extension.

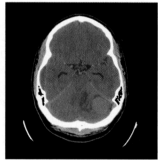

Mildly hyperdense mass in the left cerebellar hemisphere with associated surrounding white matter, vasogenic oedema and mass effect. At surgery this was confirmed to be a highly cellular medulloblastoma.

Hydrocephalus

In general, enlargement of the ventricular system may be a compensatory effect related to reduced volume of brain parenchyma seen in old age and certain neurodegenerative conditions, or hydrocephalus. Acute hydrocephalus is usually associated with signs of mass effect such as effacement of sulci and periventricular oedema (low attenuation), and may be caused by obstruction to the flow of cerebrospinal fluid somewhere along its pathway – for example, at the foramen of Monro by a colloid cyst. In this case only the ventricles upstream from the obstruction will be dilated, and in this example, only the lateral ventricles. Obstruction to the absorption of cerebrospinal fluid at the arachnoid granulations, mainly on the cerebral convexity surfaces, can result in dilation of all of the ventricles. This is known as communicating hydrocephalus. Typical causes of communicating hydrocephalus are subarachnoid haemorrhage and meningitis, and it can be confused with hydrocephalus which is caused by obstruction to outflow from the fourth ventricle.

Dural spaces

The extra-axial compartment can be subdivided into:
- Subarachnoid space (between the arachnoid and pia mater, and the basal cisterns and sulci)
- Subdural space (between the dura and arachnoid layer and includes the interhemispheric fissure and tentorium)
- Extradural space (between the dura and the inner table of the skull.)

The principal abnormality to be identified is an extra-axial haemorrhage. A subdural haematoma is usually over the cerebral convexity, but it may be located in the interhemispheric fissure, or related to the tentorium. Subdural haematomas are usually large, crescentic structures, and are often distant from the site of impact ("non-direct" or "contre-coup"). Extradural haematomas are typically related to the site of an impact, often a skull vault fracture. They are biconvex and small, limited by the vault bone sutures. The density of an extra-axial haemorrhage decreases with time. After about 12-15 days it may be isodense to brain tissue and difficult to identify. Beyond three weeks, chronic subdural haematomas are predominantly low density, occurring most often in elderly patients after minor trauma. In hyperacute haemorrhage or in patients with coagulopathy, the subdural collection may be low density, but it usually contains swirls of mixed density.

Non-haemorrhagic, low density collections of subdural fluid are important. If present acutely after trauma, they may represent cerebrospinal fluid effusions where there is a local arachnoid tear. They may have mass effect, but are usually self limiting. In the unwell, feverish patient, identifying a subdural empyema (infected subdural effusion) is critical. Its margins are usually thickened and enhance after administration of contrast. Often they may present with sinusitis.

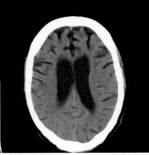

Third ventricular colloid cyst with hydrocephalus. Typical rounded hyperdense lesion at the anterior aspect of the third ventricle with dilatation of the lateral ventricles.

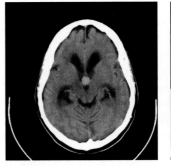

Large ventricles caused by cerebral volume loss as denoted by proportionate prominence of the frontal cerebral sulci.

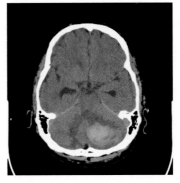

Partially haemorrhagic mass in the left cerebellar hemisphere with surrounding oedema. Because it has mass effect on the fourth ventricle, the upstream ventricular system is enlarged as shown by dilatation of the temporal horns.

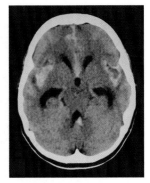

Communicating hydrocephalus with dilatation of all the ventricles in subarachnoid haemorrhage as shown by extensive high density acute blood in the subarachnoid spaces.

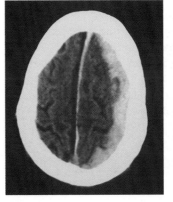

Large acute high density crescent shaped subdural haematoma over the left cerebral convexity and extending into the interhemispheric fissure.

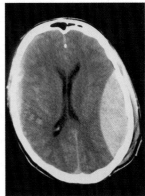

Large left acute lentiform shaped extradural haemorrhage with shallow crescentic right sided subdural haematoma and associated right cerebral contusions. Note the mild left to right subfalcine shift of the midline.

It is advisable to examine the dural venous sinuses for signs of thrombosis. In the acute setting, a thrombosed venous sinus will be expanded and hyperdense on a plain CT scan. After contrast, a filling defect denoting the thrombus may be visible.

Deciding if a lesion is intra-axial or extra-axial is an important step in the interpretation of cranial CT. The differential diagnosis is quite different for the two compartments. An extra-axial lesion will displace inwardly underlying cerebral cortex and pial blood vessels. A cerebrospinal cleft may be produced at the margin of the legion. An extra-axial lesion will often have a broad dural base or attachment, and may be associated with overlying bony changes. Some tumours are extra-axial – for example, a meningioma (a benign tumour of the meninges) is typically well defined, hyperdense, enhanced and may cause calcification. Skull vault metastases may have an extradural soft tissue component.

Eyes

- Orbital fracture (exclude muscle entrapment in blow-out fracture)
- Orbital haematoma
- Globe injury
- Optic nerve injury.

Face

- Face and foreign bodies – see chapter 13
- Check maxilla, mandible, zygoma, or pterygoid plates for fractures

Key areas for review

If, having examined the computed tomogram using the ABCs system, the study seems unremarkable, review key areas before calling the study normal.

- Always look at the scout image (scanogram). It may show a skull fracture, upper cervical spine fracture or dislocation, or incorrect positioning of the nasogastric tube.
- Re-assess for extra-axial haemorrhage. Check the periphery of each axial cut, along the falx and on the tentorium.
- Check for signs of mass effect, especially sulcal and ventricular effacement and symmetry.
- Examine the dural venous sinuses for hyperdensity and expansion on the non-enhanced CT to indicate acute thrombosis.

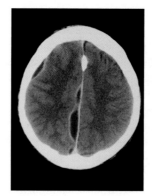

Typical appearances of a subdural empyema. Loculated cerebrospinal fluid density subdural collections over the right cerebral surface and in the interhemispheric fissure.

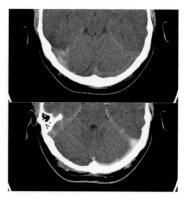

Typical appearances of thrombosis of the right lateral dural venous sinus with hyperdensity and expansion on the unenhanced image (top) and a filling defect in the sinus after contrast (bottom).

Indications for skull radiographs in trauma

- Suspected depressed skull fracture
- Foreign bodies
- Gunshot wounds
- Suspected non-accidental injury in children

Indications for non-enhanced CT in trauma*

- Glasgow Coma Scale score <13 at any time or Glasgow Coma Scale <15 two hours after injury
- Focal neurological deficit
- Seizure
- Signs of base of skull fracture
- Vomiting
- Coagulopathy
- >65 years
- Severe mechanism of injury
- Retrograde amnesia longer than 30 minutes

*Adapted from National Institute for Clinical Excellence Guidelines 2003

Head injuries

Head injuries are common. In the USA, there are over 500 000 head injuries a year, and 20% (100 000) of them have residual disabilities. About 80% are considered mild, 10% moderate, and 10% severe. Delay in diagnosis and treatment of head injuries is recognised as a major cause of preventable morbidity and mortality. Every effort should be made to accelerate the pathway to the management of these patients. Early recognition and suspicion of an intracranial injury is essential.

Plain radiography has no important role in the management of head injuries because plain radiographs provide no information on the status of the brain parenchyma. Of patients with intracranial injuries, 91% have normal skull radiographs. There are limited clinical indications for requesting plain radiography.

Trauma accounts for most cranial CT performed as an emergency, and there should be a low threshold for requesting this investigation early after trauma. Although traditionally cranial CT was reserved for patients with moderate or severe head injuries (Glasgow Coma Scale <14), there is now evidence that CT should be performed on all patients with clinical evidence of a head injury. In the United Kingdom, magnetic resonance imaging is not employed acutely, although it does have long-term applications in the investigation of cognitive or neurological deficits after head trauma.

Rapid initial imaging with CT while maintaining a low threshold for re-imaging is critical in the management of head injury patients to prevent or limit the extent of secondary brain injury.

Primary brain injury

Primary brain injury results directly from the traumatic event, the mechanism of which may be penetrating or non-penetrating (blunt). In the United Kingdom, blunt trauma to the head is far more common and, depending on the precise mechanism, can injure the brain at the point of impact (direct local coup) or distant from the point of impact (non-direct). Non-direct injuries are produced by "shear-strain" forces, which are mechanical stresses on brain tissue generated by sudden deceleration or angular rotation. Indeed, such injuries can also be produced with no direct cranial impact.

The manifestations of primary brain injury are extra-axial haemorrhage and a range of intrinsic lesions. Typically, multiple co-existing lesions are induced by direct and non-direct means.

Primary brain injury

Non-penetrating (blunt)
Direct (local impact = "coup")
- Skull fracture/scalp laceration
- Contusion
- Parenchymal haemorrhage
- Extradural haematoma
- Subdural haematoma – less commonly
- Traumatic subarachnoid haemorrhage

Non-direct
Extra-axial
- Traumatic subarachnoid haemorrhage, subdural haematoma

Intra-axial
- Cortical contusions – often called "contre-coup" injuries: They are caused by the impact of brain against rough bone or dura. The anteroinferior temporal lobes are involved in 50% of cases with cortical contusions and the anteroinferior frontal lobes are involved in 35%. They are multiple and bilateral in 90% of cases. Parasagittal and dorsolateral brainstem lesions are less common.
- Diffuse axonal injury – second most common lesion in closed head injury – 45% of cases: Typically patients present with immediate (can be transient) loss of consciousness. Diffuse axonal injury is a common cause of post-traumatic persistent coma. Multiple, usually small, white matter lesions are seen at the grey-white matter interface (mainly fronto-temporally), corpus callosum (mainly posteriorly), internal capsule and brainstem. The initial computed tomogram is normal in 50-80% of patients. Later petechial haemorrhages may develop at these sites.
- Deep cerebral and brainstem injury – associated with severe injury and a poor prognosis: Shearing of perforating arteries can lead to haemorrhaging into the basal ganglia or brainstem. CT shows hyperdense lesions of varying size with oedema.

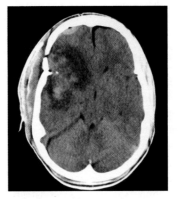 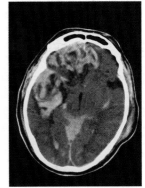

Direct partially haemorrhagic contusions in the right frontal lobe directly beneath a right frontal fracture at the site of impact. Note the small and shallow right frontal extradural haematoma.

Typical extensive indirect haemorrhagic contusions in the right frontal and temporal lobes following impact to the left parietal region as shown by soft tissue swelling over that region. Note the subdural haemorrhage layering on the tentorium and some intraventricular blood.

In general, management of cranial trauma aims to prevent or limit the degree of secondary brain injury. These injuries include ischaemia, infarction, diffuse cerebral oedema, brain herniation, and vascular complications and both contribute to and result from cyclical deterioration in local or generalised cerebral perfusion and intracranial pressure.

Meningitis

Suspected meningitis does not typically require CT before lumbar puncture. A computed tomogram is usually normal in uncomplicated meningitis. Moreover, a normal study does not exclude the possibility of brain herniation. A computed tomogram study is performed to exclude complications such as:
- Obstructive hydrocephalus
- Intraparenchymal abscess
- Subdural effusion or empyema
- Vasculitis with ischaemia/infarction
- Venous sinus thrombosis.

Imaging signs
General
- Often non-specific
- May be normal
- Signs of complications
- Subdural effusions (cerebrospinal fluid density or intensity)

Non-enhanced CT
- Mild ventricular enlargement
- Effacement of basal cisterns
- High density subarachnoid space exudates

Contrast enhanced CT
- Enhancing exudates
- Prominent pial enhancement

Subarachnoid haemorrhage

Subarachnoid haemorrhage is defined as haemorrhage into the subarachnoid space, that is, the basal cisterns, sylvian fissures, and cerebral sulci, and it can involve the intraventricular space and (rarely) interhemispheric fissure. Usually, subarachnoid haemorrhage is caused by trauma, but cerebral aneurysms (aneurysmal subarachnoid haemorrhage) are the most common non-traumatic cause.

Non-enhanced CT is the modality of choice showing high density (acute haemorrhage) in the subarachnoid space. In aneurysmal subarachnoid haemorrhage, the distribution of blood may indicate the site of the aneurysm. Non-enhanced CT is positive in 95% of acute subarachnoid haemorrhage cases within 24 hours of the ictus, but sensitivity decreases with time (<50% after a week).
Complications of subarachnoid haemorrhage:
- Early communicating hydrocephalus is typical
- Low attenuation areas in vascular distribution indicate ischaemia related to vasospasm, especially at days 4 to 10
- Late hydrocephalus (after discharge from hospital)
- Re-bleed.

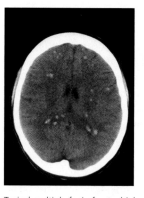

Typical multiple foci of petechial haemorrhage in diffuse axonal injury with high density lesions in the fronto-temporal regions mainly at the grey-white interface, and also in the posterior corpus callosum.

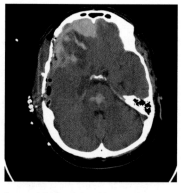

Severe right frontal and temporal traumatic injuries. There is a focal haemorrhage in the pons which is a poor prognostic sign.

Indications for non-enhanced CT in meningitis

- Reduced level of consciousness
- Signs of raised intracranial pressure
- Focal neurological deficit
- Seizures
- Immunocompromised status

Consider contrast enhanced CT in this situation

Imaging guidelines for subarachnoid haemorrhage

Non-enhanced CT
- If non-enhanced CT positive – CT angiography or catheter angiography
- If CT angiography positive – surgery or catheter angiography and endovascular coiling
- If CT angiography negative – catheter angiography
- If catheter angiography positive – surgery or endovascular coiling
- If catheter angiography negative:
  - if vasospasm, large haematoma, index of suspicion – repeat catheter angiography at 2 weeks
  - magnetic resonance image for superficial parenchymal lesion – for example, cavernous angioma
  - if no vasospasm or probable venous bleed – no further investigation or repeat CT angiography at 2 weeks
  - If non-enhanced computed tomogram is negative, advise lumbar puncture

Stroke

The term stroke refers to a cerebrovascular accident and includes ischaemic and haemorrhagic aetiologies. In this section, we discuss the CT imaging of acute ischaemic stroke.

Causes of ischaemic stroke:

- Embolic phenomena from cardiac source (15-20% of all ischaemic strokes) – for example, atrial fibrillation, and extracranial arterial source (typically atheroma in carotid bulb)
- Narrowing of extracranial carotid arteries → watershed (borderzone) ischaemia caused by hypoperfusion
- Thrombosis or narrowing of major intracranial arteries (for example, acute middle cerebral artery thrombosis)
- Small vessel vasculopathy (secondary to ageing, diabetes, hypertension or vasculitis).

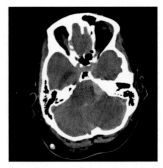

Subarachnoid haemorrhage with an acute inferior anterior interhemispheric clot as is typical with an anterior communicating artery aneurysm.

Acute subarachnoid haemorrhage in the left cerebello-pontine angle, fourth ventricle and lateral aspect of the medulla as is typical with an aneurysm at the origin of the posterior inferior cerebellar artery.

Vascular territory infarct

Imaging
Hyperacute (<24 hours after ictus)

- Non-enhanced CT normal in 50-60%
- Hyperdense proximal middle cerebral artery in 35-50%
- Early mass effect – sulcal effacement
- Loss of conspicuity of lentiform nucleus
- Loss of grey-white matter differentiation – insular ribbon lost

Imaging guidelines for stroke

If not for thrombolysis
Non-enhanced CT

- Within 24 hours to exclude non–ischaemic cause (for example, tumour or haemorrhage)
- Acutely: if high risk of haemorrhage (hypertension, low platelet count, clotting disorder, or anticoagulation therapy)
  - Subsequent fall in Glasgow Coma Scale score may indicate haemorrhagic transformation
  - Would preclude anticoagulation treatment or thrombolysis
- Carry out non-enhanced CT acutely, within three hours if thrombolysis considered

Acute (1-3 days after ictus)

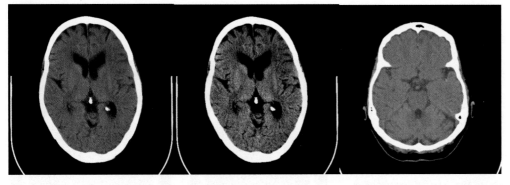

Acute left MCA territory infarct with subtle low attenuation in the inferior left frontal lobe on the normal cerebral window setting (left) and on the more conspicuous stroke window setting (middle). Note in the right hand figure the dense left middle cerebral artery in the sylvian fissure, in keeping with a thrombus.

- Non-enhanced CT region of low attenuation involving grey and white matter
- Increasing mass effect
- Haemorrhagic transformation
  - Caused by reperfusion because of embolus breakdown or collateral flow
  - Rarely before 24-48 hours, it occurs in 20% of cases and mainly involves basal ganglia and cortex
  - Increased risk with thromboembolic infarct, diabetes, or thrombolysis and with very early hypodensity on CT

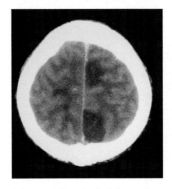

Subacute infarcts in the left anterior cerebral artery territory.

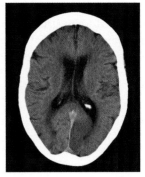

Subacute infarct in the left posterior cerebral artery territory.

Subacute (3-10 days after ictus)
- Non-enhanced CT

  Wedge shaped area of low attenuation – well defined

  Mass effect peaks at about seven days
- Contrast enhanced CT

  Parenchymal enhancement – gyriform. Due to breakdown of blood-brain barrier

Chronic (>14 days after isctus)
- Non-enhanced CT

  Encephalomalacia develops

  Volume loss – sulcal and ventricular enlargement

  No mass effect

  Wallerian degeneration – ipsilateral midbrain atrophy

  Contralateral cerebellar atrophy

  Enhancement can persist for up to two months

  Dystrophic calcification can occur

Intraparenchymal haemorrhage

It is important to differentiate a primary haemorrhage from a haemorrhage that is caused by an underlying lesion, specifically a tumour. Trauma remains the most common cause of parenchymal haemorrhage, and, in non-traumatic cases, often the patient has a history of hypertension. Haemorrhage within a primary or secondary brain tumour usually evolves in a different pattern where there is persistent mass effect and surrounding oedema, possibly recurrent or multifocal haemorrhage and areas of enhancement after contrast administration. A delayed computed tomogram before and after contrast or magnetic resonance imaging is often necessary after two months when the haemorrhage has resolved. CT or catheter angiography may be indicated acutely if an underlying vascular malformation is suspected and surgery is planned immediately.

Hypertensive haemorrhage

Hypertensive heamorrhage is the most common cause of parenchymal haemorrhage in elderly patients with hypertension.

On non-contrast enhanced CT, the typical appearances are of a high density mass in the striato-capsular region (in 65% of presentations). Haemorrhage in the thalamus occurs in 20%, although the brainstem, cerebellum and periphery of the cerebral hemispheres is more uncommon. There is often intraventricular extension and evidence of a background of hypertension. In particular, there may be evidence of small vessel disease with low attenuation lesions in the cerebral white matter, brainstem, basal ganglia, thalami, and cerebellum.

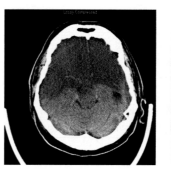

Bilateral anterior circulation territory stroke due to strangulation.

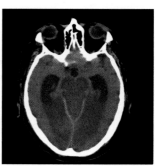

Bilateral and complete posterior circulation infarct after hanging and bilateral vertebral artery occlusion.

Causes of intraparenchymal haemorrhage

Trauma

Non-trauma

In elderly patients
- Hypertension
- Amyloid angiopathy
- Haemorrhagic transformation in an infarct
- Haemorrhagic tumour
- Coagulopathy

Younger adults
- Underlying vascular abnormality (including aneurysm or arteriovenous malformation)
- Venous sinus thrombosis
- Vasculitis
- Haemorrhagic encephalitis
- Cavernoma

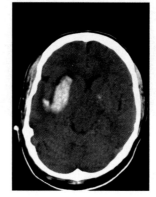

Typical acute hypertensive haemorrhage in the right basal ganglia.

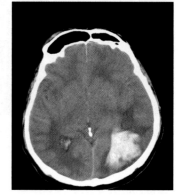

Hypertensive encephalopathy. Acute haemorrhage in the left parieto-occipital region on a background of marked cerebral swelling and symmetric posterior predominantly white matter low attenuation.

Imaging signs

- Non-enhanced CT
- High density mass
- Typically striato-capsular (60–65% of hypertensive patients)
- Thalamus (20% of hypertensive patients), pons and cerebellum (10% of hypertensive patients), lobar 5–10% of hypertensive patients
- With or without intraventricular extension
- Mass effect
- Hydrocephalus due to mass effect
- Evidence of hypertensive small vessel disease with low attenuation lesions in the central white matter, basal ganglia or thalami

---

KEY POINTS

- Skull radiographs are not indicated in head injury
- Delayed management of head injuries is a major cause of preventable morbidity and mortality in patients who have experienced trauma
- Use a systematic assessment to make an accurate diagnosis
- It is important to maintain a low threshold for performing, or even repeating, a computed tomogram head examination in the trauma setting.

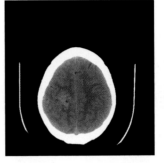
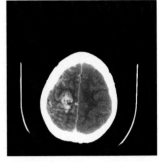

Arteriovenous malformation in the right fronto-parietal region with an ill defined high density lesion with little mass effect on unenhanced images but which enhances avidly following contrast.

Arteriovenous malformation in the right fronto-parietal region with serpiginous tubular structures in keeping with abnormal vessels.

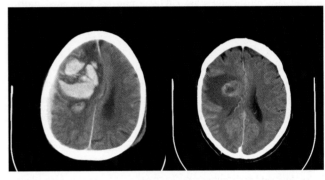

Acute haemorrhagic mass in the right frontal lobe with associated oedema and mass effect (left). The right-hand delayed contrast enhanced computed tomogram shows the same patient a few weeks later and shows an underlying peripherally enhancing mass, which was found to be a melanoma metastasis.

CHAPTER 13

Face

Simon Holmes, Laurence H Berman, Otto Chan

The face is often injured in road traffic crashes, fights, and assaults. Up to 70% of people who are in road traffic crashes sustain facial injuries, and most of these are soft tissue injuries. Associated injuries occur in up to half of patients with facial fractures, but, surprisingly, only 2% of these associated injuries occur to the cervical spine. The distribution of injuries to the face varies with patient population, but the injuries usually occur to the midface or mandible.

Accurate radiological diagnosis is central to the management of maxillofacial trauma and other medical and surgical conditions that affect the facial bones. Although computed tomography is used increasingly in emergency assessment of such patients, plain radiographs play a central role in the initial management.

Cervical spine injury should be excluded before patients are positioned for plain radiographs to avoid causing secondary neurological injury. Patients are imaged best while they are standing up, to maximise diagnostic yield from plain films. This may be impossible, however, because of the patient's other injuries and their level of consciousness or intoxication.

Studying the air-bone interfaces, cortical continuity, and symmetry helps the non-specialist to assess the facial bones.

Anatomy

The key to interpretation of imaging of maxillofacial injuries is to understand the basic anatomy and the radiological appearances of the face. The face can be divided into three areas:
- Midface (maxilla, zygoma, and nasal bones)
- Above midface (orbit and frontal sinuses)
- Below midface (mandible).

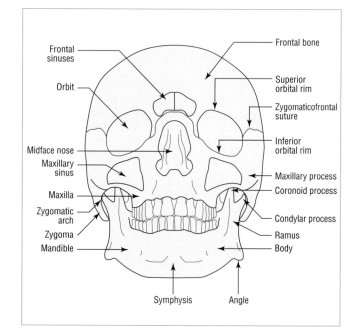

Anatomy of the face.

Recommended radiological views for facial injuries

- Midface and orbital floor – occipitomental and occipitomental 30°
- Zygomatic arch – occipitomental and submentovertex
- Mandible – orthopantomogram and posteroanterior and lateral oblique
- Orbit – occipitomental and posteroanterior 20°
- Frontal sinuses – posteroanterior 20° and lateral
- Nasal bone – none usually or coned lateral

ABCs systematic assessment

- **A**dequacy: choose correct view and have a low threshold to request computed tomography
- **A**lignment: check Dolan's lines, McGrigor's lines, and Campbell's lines
- **B**one: check all the bones in the midface and above and below the midface
- **C**artilage and joints: check the zygomaticofrontal sutures and temporomandibular joints
- **S**inuses: check for opacification and polyps, and check for the presence of an air-fluid level
- **S**oft tissues: look for soft tissue swelling and surgical/orbital emphysema. Check for foreign bodies.

Adequacy

The standard radiographs needed for the evaluation of facial injuries will depend on the clinical findings and suspected injuries. Standard views are the occipitomental and occipitomental 30° views. Although most textbooks recommend a lateral radiograph for facial injuries, it is rarely helpful and has been discarded as a routine view. It is important to obtain good quality radiographs in an emergency situation, although this is not always possible because patients can be uncooperative, intoxicated, or unconscious.

Most midfacial injuries are complex and the threshold for computed tomography should be low to confirm or refute the diagnosis. With thin-section multidetector computed tomography, exquisite detail for bony and soft tissue injuries can be obtained. Multiplanar and three dimensional reconstructions can be done in seconds and using relatively low doses.

Alignment and bones

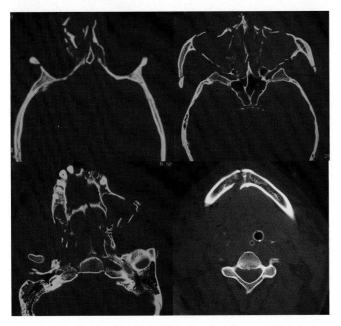

Computed tomograms with LeFort II fracture and midline separation. Level of nasion (arrows) (top left), level of maxillary antrum (arrows) (top right), level of hard palate (arrows) (bottom left), and level of chin (symphysis menti) (arrows) (bottom right).

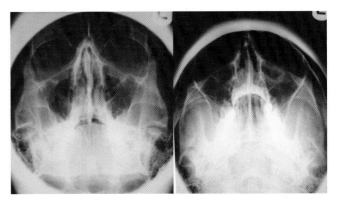

Occipitomental (left), and occipitomental 30° views (right).

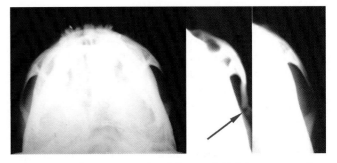

Magnified view showing zygomatic arch fracture (left). Submentovertex view (middle) magnified to show zygomatic arch (right).

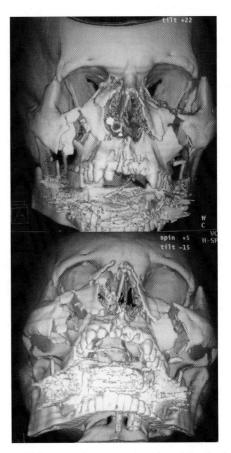

Three dimensional reconstruction – frontal view (top), occipitomental view (bottom).

Occipitomental view

Dolan described three lines that resemble an elephant's head and trunk. This is a helpful way of initially evaluating the occipitomental view.

Several other lines can be used to trace and look for steps, lines, breaks, and changes of contour between the two sides.

- McGrigor's line 1 – starts lateral to the right zygomaticofrontal suture. Check that the zygomaticofrontal suture is not wider than the opposite side, and then that the line goes up the superior orbital ridge, across the opposite side, and out through the contralateral zygomaticofrontal suture.
- McGrigor's line 2 – starts at the superior and lateral aspect of the right zygomatic arch, runs medially to the infraorbital margin, over the contour of the nose, and across the other side.
- McGrigor's line 3 – begins on the inferior and lateral surface of the zygomatic arch and moves medially. At the floor of the maxillary antrum, it goes across the alveolar process and repeats the movement across the other side.
- Campbell's line 4 – runs along the medial aspect of the coronoid process inferomedially and across the superior surface of the body and ramus of the mandible. Finally, it crosses the midline over the superior surface of the symphysis menti and goes across the other side.
- Campbell's line 5 – follows the inferior surface of the mandible from the lateral aspect of the right lateral condylar process to the angle of the mandible and along the inferior surface of the mandible, across the midline to the left condylar process.

When drawing these lines across the entire face, note any lucencies or sclerotic areas of the bones that cross or breach the cortex. These are often fractures. In particular, check the zygomatic arch and all the individual bones that make up the face. Fractures of the face are particularly hard to detect because several bony structures overlap.

Orthopantomograms

Check:

- The lower border by examining the air-bone interface, looking for cortical discontinuity from left condyle to right condyle.
- For broken or missing teeth. Any missing teeth raise the possibility of aspiration by the patient. Dental pathologies can be diagnosed at this time. They can be important for the ongoing management of traumatic injuries.
- The cortical outline of the inferior alveolar canal. Step deformities often result in cortical disruption.
- Dental occlusion – spacing between the upper and lower teeth should be equal. Often a condylar neck fracture with shortening of the posterior face can be picked up in this way.
- The rest of the film – valuable information about maxillary and mandibular pathologies and dental injuries should be obtained.

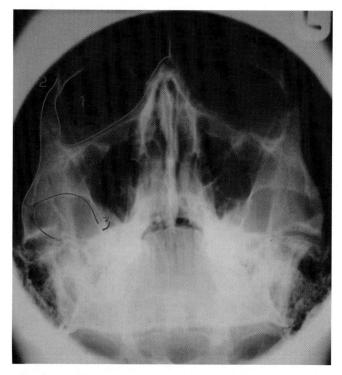

Dolan's lines look like an elephant's head.

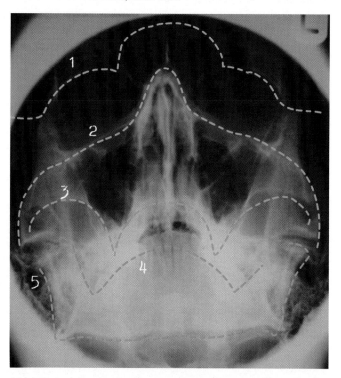

Occipitomental view showing McGrigor's lines (blue), and Campbell's lines (green).

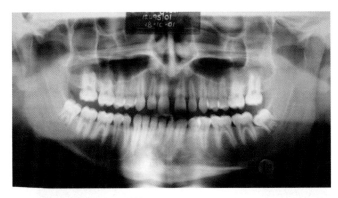

Orthopantomogram of mandible.

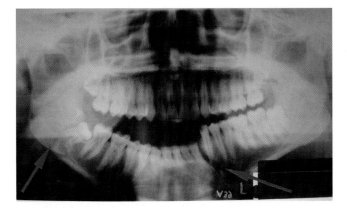

Orthopantomogram showing two large fractures of mandible (arrows).

Diagnostic pitfalls when assessing orthopantomograms

- Fracture at the angle of mandible can be imitated by air in the oropharynx. It is important to show that any cortical disruption extends no further than the edge of the bone
- Symphyseal fractures can be imitated by superimposition of the cervical vertebra on the midline of the mandible

Fractures of the mandible

These injuries are common and are the result of moderate energy transfer to the lower face. Fractures typically occur at sites of weakness or at sites of bony pathology. The mandible is a rigid ring that is similar to the pelvis, therefore if you see one fracture, always look for a second. The orthopantomogram may not clearly show the midline fractures, so a posteroanterior mandible view is always performed as well.

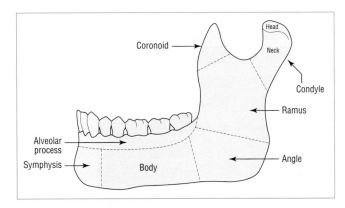

Anatomy of the mandible.

Condylar fractures and temporomandibular joint injuries can be difficult to identify, and further views may be necessary.

The symptoms for fractures of the mandible are subjective alteration in bite, pain, swelling, paraesthesia or anaesthesia of inferior alveolar nerve, or inability to open the mouth after a history of trauma. The signs of a fractured mandible are deranged occlusion, bony pain, paraesthesia, crepitus, bleeding from the ear, and sublingual haematoma.

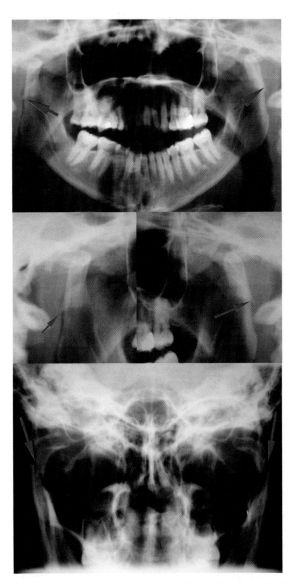

Orthopantomogram with angulated and displaced fractures of both condyles (top). Magnified view with a fracture of the neck of the right condyle (middle left). Magnified view with a fracture of the neck of the left condyle (middle right). Towne's view confirms displaced and angulated fractures of the neck of both condyles (arrows in bottom orthopantomomogram).

Fractures of the mandible

Anatomical site	Cause of weakness	Radiological view
Condyle	Anatomically thin	Orthopantomogram Posteroanterior mandible Lateral oblique Towne's view
Angle	Unerupted third molar	Orthopantomogram Posteroanterior mandible
Parasymphysis	Long canine root	Orthopantomogram Posteroanterior mandible
Body	Trauma	Orthopantomogram Posteroanterior mandible
Symphysis	Trauma Fall on chin Direct blow	Orthopantomogram Posteroanterior mandible Lower mandibular occlusal
Pathological fracture	Cysts, infection, tumour, others	Orthopantomogram Posteroanterior mandible Computed tomography scan

Middle third facial fractures

These injuries are classified into several anatomically based fractures.

Middle third facial fractures

Central
- Nasal
- Nasoethnoid
- Maxilliary – LeFort I, II, and III

Lateral
- Zygomatic

Nasal fractures are diagnosed clinically. Maxillary fractures are classified by LeFort lines. In practice, the precise characterisation of these injuries is difficult and not of major importance in the emergency room. Mixed fracture configuration patterns are common.

The symptoms and signs of middle third fractures are epistaxis, diplopia, swelling, infraorbital nerve anaesthesia or paraesthesia, deranged occlusion, subconjunctival haematoma, facial asymmetry, and mobile or missing teeth.

LeFort injuries

Rene LeFort was a French doctor who studied facial injuries in cadavers. He dropped heads from a height and then described patterns of facial injuries. All LeFort injuries require plain imaging and computed tomography to determine the extent, distribution, and pattern of the injuries before further management is attempted

- LeFort I: a fracture above the alveolar process, which leads to the alveolar process being separated from the rest of the maxilla. Clinically, the upper teeth can be moved away from the nose.
- LeFort II: the fracture line extends above the nose. In theory, the upper teeth and nose can be moved en bloc away from the rest of the face.
- LeFort III: the face is separated from the rest of the head (craniofacial dissociation).

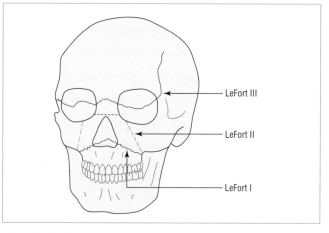

Posteroanterior view of mandible with two large fractures (arrows).

LeFort III
LeFort II
LeFort I

LeFort classification.

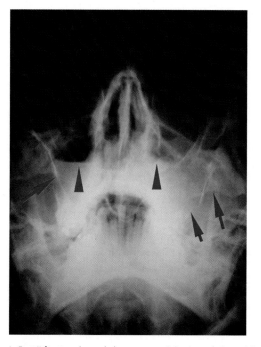

LeFort II fracture (arrow) shown on occipitomental view with air-fluid levels seen in both maxillary sinuses (arrowheads).

Most of these injuries do not usually present with a straightforward symmetrical injury, and combination injuries are common. The final classification, however, is made on the basis of the highest injury.

Tripod fractures

These are the most common facial fractures and usually result from a blow to the cheek and direct injury of the zygoma. The fracture involves the frontal process of the zygoma, the zygomatic arch, and the maxillary process (superior and lateral wall of the maxillary antrum) – hence tripod fracture. Diagnosis is simple with standard occipitomental and occipitomental 30° views. Soft tissue swelling, an air-fluid level, and some rotation (best seen on computed tomography) are often present.

Orbital injuries

These injuries are classified by the site of involvement.
- Orbital rim
- Orbital floor
- Medial wall
- Lateral wall

The symptoms and signs of orbital injuries include ecchymosis, subconjunctival haemorrhage, diplopia, enophthalmos, and infraorbital anaesthesia or paraesthesia.

Blow out fractures

These are injuries sustained by a direct blow to the eyeball, which then breaks either the floor or medial wall of the orbit, not the orbital rim. Herniation of some contents may occur, particularly of retro-orbital fat associated with depression of the orbital floor. The inferior rectus muscle can sometimes be trapped, or it may herniate with the fat. This may lead to enophthalmos and diplopia on upward gaze and numbness over the inferior orbital margin. Urgent surgical referral is advised. Radiologically, the classic appearances are those of a teardrop on the roof of the maxillary antrum. Some other orbital wall fractures and orbit injuries are usually investigated best with plain radiography or ultrasonography initially. Computed tomography, however, is often invaluable.

Upper third facial fractures

These are unusual injuries and include fractures of the frontal bone, extended nasoethmoidal fractures, and supraorbital injuries.

Epistaxis, soft tissue swelling, deformity, cerebrospinal fluid rhinorrhoea, anaesthesia of infraorbital nerve, and pain on upward gaze.

Accurate diagnosis is essential for upper facial third fractures. Precise information about fractures of the frontal sinus with respect to anterior and posterior walls is key to management. For this reason, computed tomography scans (axial, coronal, and three dimensional reconstructions) are invariably required in these cases, particularly if any signs of retrobulbar haemorrhage are present (proptosis, pain, ophthalmoplegia, and diminishing visual acuity).

Indirect signs of orbital trauma

- Soft tissue swelling
- Surgical/orbital emphysema
- Opaque sinuses
- Air-fluid levels in the sinuses
- Teardrop sign

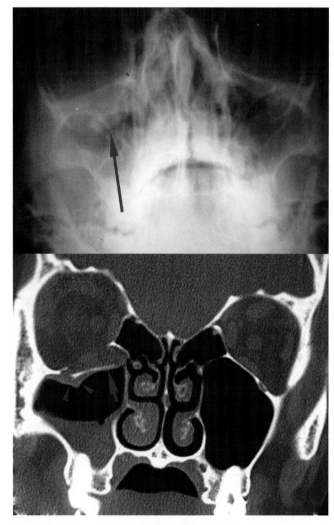

Teardrop in right maxillary antrum on occipitomental view (arrow) (top). Coronal computed tomogram (bottom) shows a small depressed fracture of the floor of the right orbit (arrows), some soft tissue protruding into the roof of the right maxillary antrum (arrowheads), and a swollen and trapped inferior rectus (arrow).

Cartilage and joints

The zygomaticofrontal sutures should be of equal size, and the condylar processes should lie in the temporomandibular joint, especially on the orthopantomogram and lateral oblique views.

Sinuses and soft tissues

Asymmetry of the face is an extremely helpful finding, particularly asymmetry of the soft tissues, air-fluid levels in the sinuses, mucosal thickening, and soft tissue masses (teardrops and polyps) seen in the sinuses. Also, look for radio-opaque foreign bodies, particularly glass and metal.

Swelling of the soft tissue indicates site of injury. Look at the soft tissues by blocking out the lower half of the face from the infra-orbital margin, and then repeat the exercise and check the lower half, in particular looking for fluid levels and teardrops in the maxillary sinuses and soft tissue swelling over the face or infraorbital margin.

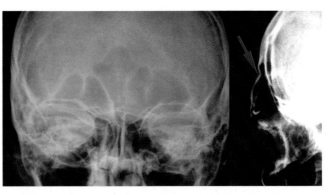

Anteroposterior view shows a subtle fracture line (left). Lateral view confirms a depressed fracture of the anterior margin of the frontal sinus (arrow) (right).

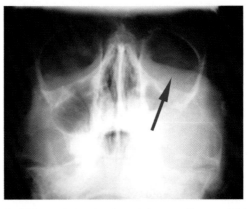

Occipitomental view showing soft tissue swelling over left infraorbital margin (arrows).

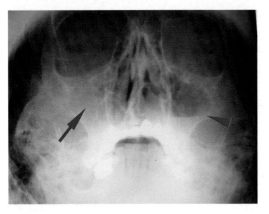

Opaque right maxillary antrum (arrow) and air-fluid level in left maxillary antrum (arrowhead).

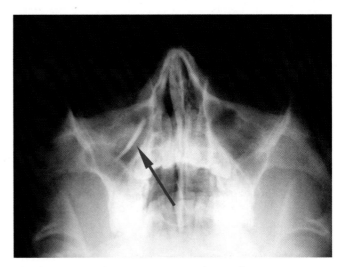

Glass fragment (arrow) seen on occipitomental view only.

ABCs systematic assessment

Adequacy
- Use correct view for plain radiographs and request computed tomography when necessary

Alignment
- Check Dolan's, McGrigor's, and Campbell's lines

Bones
- Check all bones in the midface and upper and lower third of the face.

Cartilage and joints
- Check the zygomaticofrontal sutures and temporomandibular joints

Sinuses and soft tissues
- Check for local swelling of the soft tissue, surgical/orbital emphysema, air-fluid levels and opaque sinuses, teardrop injuries, foreign bodies such as glass and metal

KEY POINTS

- Understand anatomy and classification of injuries
- Facial injuries (usually soft tissue injuries) are common
- Plain radiographs play a central role in the initial assessment
- Always look for a second fracture in the mandible
- Computed tomography shows exquisitely detailed anatomy and the extent and distribution of injury.

CHAPTER 14

Cervical Spine

Clint W Sliker, Kathirkamanathan Shanmuganathan

Fractures of the cervical spine are potentially devastating injuries that require prompt diagnosis and stabilisation to minimise the risk and severity of associated neurological injury. The pattern, frequency, and distribution of these injuries vary with the population studied. In adults, injuries typically affect C1-2 and C5-6. Cervical spine injury in children is less common, with the upper cervical spine usually involved. Up to 40% of cervical spine injuries are associated with neurological injury with 5-10% reported as the result of missed injury, and consequent lack of cervical stabilisation. About 0.1% of injuries of the cervical spinal cord do not present with a radiographic abnormality. Such spinal cord injuries without radiological abnormalities typically affect those people with prominent cervical spine degenerative disease, but they may be seen in young paediatric patients.

Anatomy

A rudimentary understanding of the anatomy of the cervical spine is necessary to analyse cervical spine radiographs. The cervical spine is comprised of seven bony segments (each segment is made of two components: the vertebral body and the neural arches), ligamentous connections, and intervertebral discs.

Vertebrae C2 to C7 are similar morphologically. Fibrocartilaginous intervertebral discs connect the vertebral bodies. Each vertebral body joins a vertebral neural arch that is comprised of bilateral pedicles, facets, and laminae with a single posterior spinous process. They form a protective cage, the spinal canal, around the spinal cord. Small lateral transverse processes transmit the vertebral arteries via the foramina transversarium (C6-2).

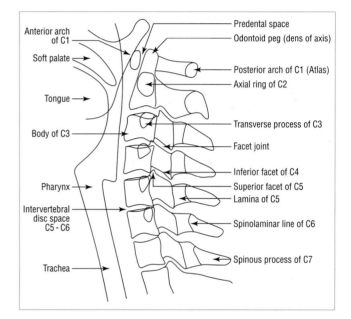

Anatomy of cervical spine.

The axial ring is the ring-like structure projecting over the C2 vertebral body on lateral projection. It represents summation of the shadow of the C2 vertebral body and lateral masses

The C2 (axis) is distinguished from the adjacent levels by a superiorly directed anterior protruberance, the odontoid process or dens, which articulates with C1.

The ring-like C1 (atlas) does not have a true body and it articulates with C2 and the base of the skull via bilateral lateral masses. No C1-2 intervertebral disc exists. The atlantodental joint is anterior.

Spinal stability depends mainly on the integrity of soft tissue structures. Of these, the ligaments are of greatest importance. The major longitudinal ligaments are the anterior longitudinal ligament, posterior longitudinal ligament, and ligamentum flavum. The supra and interspinous ligaments connect the spinous processes. Tough capsules join the interfacet joints. The transverse ligament spans the interval between C1 lateral masses posterior to the dens.

ABCs systematic assessment

- **A**dequacy
- **A**lignment
- **B**one
- **C**artilage and joints
- **S**oft tissues

Adequacy

If the patient is fully conscious, has no distracting injuries, no symptoms, and no clinical signs, then no imaging is necessary. The traditional acute trauma series comprises three views: the lateral, the anteroposterior, and the open mouth odontoid (peg) views. Lateral radiographs show most injuries.

> **Radiological projections and adequate anatomical coverage**
>
> - Lateral view: must include from the base of skull to T1 superior endplate
> - Anteroposterior radiograph: entire C3 vertebral body to T1 and the C2 spinous process should be visible
> - Open mouth odontoid view: C1 and C2 margins should be visible

Interpretation of lateral radiographs

Adequacy

The base of the skull to the T1 superior vertebral body should be seen clearly. Overlap is limited because of restricted rotation. Cortical and trabecular detail are clear. The prevertebral shadow is shown. The lower cervical spine should not be obscured by overlying anatomy (shoulders) or extrinsic structures (jewellery or monitoring devices). If the C7-T1 junction cannot be seen, repeat the film. If it is still not visible further imaging is needed.

> **Always review lateral views with the spinous processes oriented in the same direction as the computed tomography sagittal reconstructions and magnetic resonance imaging performed at your institution**

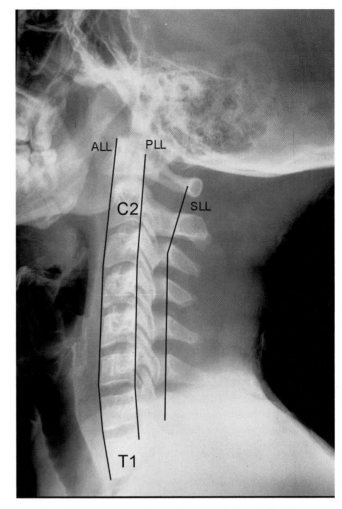

Lines of cervical spine on a lateral view. (ALL=anterior longitudinal ligament line, PLL=posterior longitudinal ligament line, SLL=spinolaminar longitudinal ligament line). The SLL may deviate posteriorly between C1 and C3.

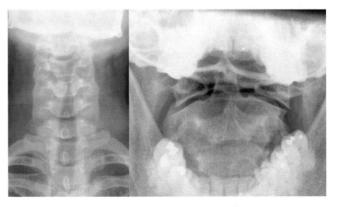

Anteroposterior radiograph of normal cervical spine (left), and open mouth odontoid view (right).

Alignment

Unless pathologically ossified or calcified, the ligaments are invisible on radiographs. Carefully follow the anterior longitudinal ligament line, the posterior longitudinal ligament line, and the spinolaminar ligament line. Search for any abrupt alterations in alignment, which may infer ligamentous injury and instability. If signs of instability are present, an injury should be considered unstable until the patient and radiographs are evaluated together by a specialist.

Normally, a gentle lordosis (a gradual curve convex anteriorly) is seen. Loss of the lordosis is not uncommon in trauma patients for a variety of reasons, such as pain, spasm, cervical collar, supine position, degenerative changes. Fusion can be caused by congenital variants (such as Klippel-Feil), inflammation, or after surgery or infection.

A hyperflexion sprain presents with a focally reverse lordosis (a kyphosis) that is usually accompanied by fanning (abrupt widening of the interlaminar space), which indicates injury to the posterior ligament complex. Facet subluxation may be manifested by focal uncovering of the articular surfaces and anterior displacement of the more superior facet.

Unilateral facet dislocation results in anterior displacement of the vertebral body by less than one half of the vertebral body's width. The dislocated facet is displaced anteriorly, and the levels above the site of the injury may take on a "bow tie" configuration as a result of associated rotation.

Bilateral facet dislocation is characterised by dislocation of the anterior vertebral body by more than half of the vertebral body's width. The intervertebral disc space is narrowed, with little, if any, rotation shown.

Alignment

- Anterior longitudinal line should be symmetric
- Posterior longitudinal line should be symmetric
- Spinolaminar lines: there should be a gradual offset C1 to C3
- Interlaminar spaces should be symmetrical
- Predental space – should be ≤3 mm in an adult and ≤5 mm in a child

Bone

Inspect the vertebrae using the same starting point at every level. The cortex and trabeculae should be defined; no discontinuity, angulation, step off, bowing, or abrupt alteration in density should be seen. No fragment should project over the spinal canal.

Dens (odontoid) fractures are divided into three subtypes, each with distinct radiographic presentation. For simplicity, also they can be classified into high or low dens fractures.

A high dens fracture usually involves the middle and lower dens. Clear disruption is diagnostic. Abnormal odontoid angulation (normal 10-20° relative to C2 body long axis) infers a fracture.

Types of dens fractures

- Type I: Occurs at the odontoid tip. It is rare, and is a high dens fracture
- Type II: Runs from body to base of dens. It is a high dens fracture
- Type III: Low dens fracture extending into C2 body

Mechanisms of injury to the cervical spine

- Hyperflexion
- Hyperextension
- Rotation
- Axial compression
- Distraction
- Lateral bending/shearing
- Complex or combined vectors

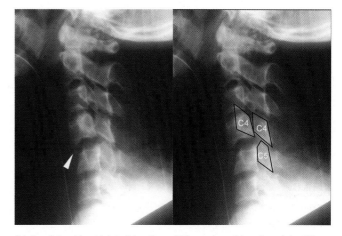

C4-5 unilateral facet joint dislocation – 20° anterior subluxation of the C4 vertebral body (arrowheads) (left), and C4 and C5 facets outlined (right). Rotation above the injury accounts for the bow tie sign at C3 and C4.

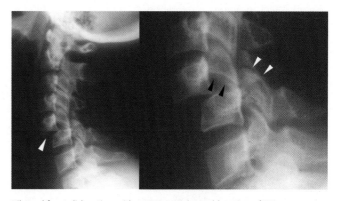

Bilateral facet dislocation with a 75% anteriror subluxation of C5 (arrowhead,) (left). Magnified view on right shows bare facet articular surfaces (arrowheads).

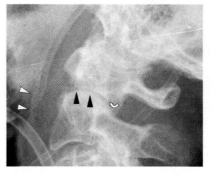

High dens fracture (type II) – lateral magnified view shows fracture at the odontoid base (black arrowheads), with posterior cortical step off (curved arrow) and prevertebral soft tissue swelling (white arrowheads).

A clearly defined fracture through the base of the odontoid with C2 body extension renders the diagnosis of a low dens fracture straightforward. Subtle signs of a low dens fracture are disruption of the axial ring and C2 vertebral body width greater than that of C3.

Traumatic spondylolysis of C2, the hangman's fracture, is characterised by disruption of the pars interarticularis region, which is situated between the C1-2 and C2-3 interfacet joints. The hyperextension teardrop fracture typically affects the C2 vertebral body. It is distinguished by a small, triangular (teardrop) fragment at the anterior inferior vertebral body.

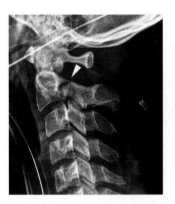 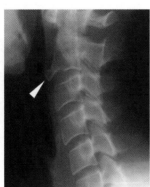

Hangman's fracture (arrowhead at pars fracture).

Hyperextension teardrop fracture (arrowhead).

When the posterior vertebral body height is 3 mm more than the anterior vertebral body height, a compression fracture is diagnosed. Typically, an anterior cortical defect or a wedge-like deformity is present. When posterior vertebral body fragment retropulsion is also present, it is considered a burst fracture. A large inferior teardrop fragment with posterior displacement of the main vertebral body fragment indicates a hyperflexion teardrop fracture. Usually, posterior displacement compromises the spinal canal. The spinous processes may fracture at any level. At the C6, C7, and T1 levels, the fracture is also known as a clay shoveler's fracture.

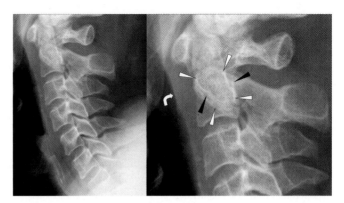

Low dens fracture (type III). Lateral magnified view (right) shows subtle buckling (black arrowheads) of the C2 axial ring (white arrowhead) with prevertebral soft tissue swelling (curved arrow).

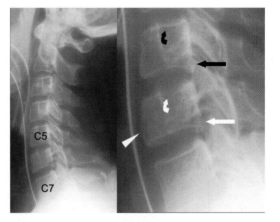

Subtle C6 burst fracture, without (left) and with (right) magnification. Anterior vertebral body cortical bowing (white arrowhead), inferior posterior fragment retropulsion (white arrow), and ill defined superior endplate (white curved arrow). Note the well defined C5 superior endplate (black curved arrow) and posterior cortex (black arrow).

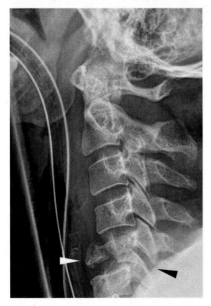

C5 hyperflexion teardrop fracture (white arrowhead), with posterior vertebral body translation and C5-6 interfacet diastasis (black arrowhead).

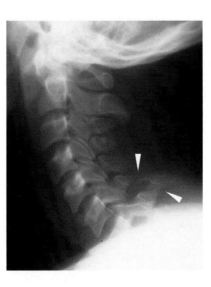

C6 and C7 clay shoveler's fractures (arrowheads).

The spinolaminar interval (space between the spinolaminar line and the posterior facet margins) alters when a traumatically isolated articular pillar, with or without an intrinsic pillar fracture, is present. An abrupt transition between levels occurs.

Cartilage and joints

The intervertebral discs may be involved in many injury patterns. Degenerative narrowing should be symmetric; a widened space is abnormal. Facet margins should be parallel, and incongruity should prompt scrutiny of the affected segment for other signs of injury, such as fanning.

A hyperextension dislocation may be extremely subtle. Typically, the affected intervertebral disc is asymmetric. The levels above the injury may be displaced posteriorly with associated widening of the interfacet joints (normal ≤2 mm).

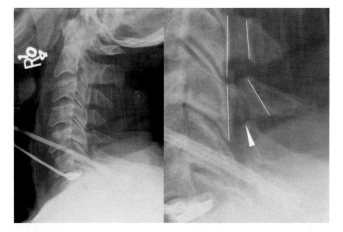

C5 isolated articular pillar (left) and magnified view (right). Note the asymmetry of the C5 spinolaminar interval compared with the superior levels (intervals demarcated by white lines) and bone fragment in C5 interval (arrowhead).

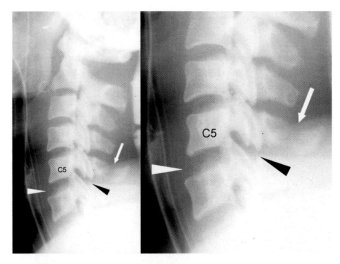

A C5-6 hyperextension dislocation with wide C5-6 intervertebral disc space (white arrowheads), C5 posterior translocation, wide C5-6 interfacet joints (black arrowheads), and C5 spinous process fracture (white arrow).

Atlanto-occipital dissociation indicates disruption of the junction of the skull and spine. An abnormal basiodental interval indicates injury, but this may be falsely normal. A more sensitive sign is an abnormal posterior axial interval.

The predental space is the interval between the posterior cortex of the C1 anterior arch and the anterior cortex of the dens. In adults, it should measure ≤3 mm, whereas in children, it should measure no more than 5 mm. Enlargement indicates transverse ligament insufficiency.

Atlanto-occipital relation

- Basiodental interval – distance between the tip of clivus (basion) and the tip of dens
- Posterior axial interval – perpendicular distance between the basion and posterior axial line. Posterior axial line represents cranial extension of posterior longitudinal line

Normal measurements
- Basiodental interval: ≤12 mm
- Posterior axial interval: <12 mm when basion anterior to posterior axial line; <4 mm when posterior to posterior axial line

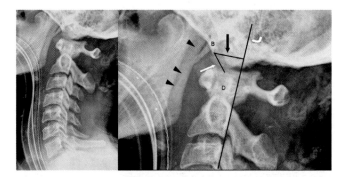

Atlanto-occipital dissociation with magnification (right), showing an abnormal posterior axial interval (black arrow), basiodental interval (white arrow), and prevertebral soft tissue swelling (arrowheads). Posterior axial line (curved arrow) (B=basion, D=dens).

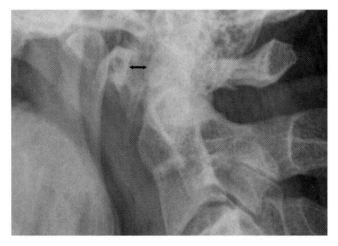

Widened predental space, 6 mm (double arrow) on lateral radiograph suggests a torn transverse ligament.

Soft tissues

A normal prevertebral soft tissue shadow does not exclude an injury. An abnormal prevertebral soft tissue shadow (secondary to haemorrhage) may be the only indicator of an injury, although other causes of this appearance exist. The thickness and the contour of the shadow should be evaluated. The airway and pharynx should be checked for swallowed foreign bodies, teeth, and malpositioned life support devices.

Interpretation of anteroposterior radiographs

Adequacy

Vertebrae C3-T1 should be seen. Endotracheal and oropharyngeal tubes should not obscure vertebrae.

Alignment

The spinous processes should be in a line. If the patient is rotated, they may lose a strict vertical orientation, but symmetric relations are maintained. Abrupt alteration in alignment indicates injury, such as unilateral facet dislocation.

Bone

The aforementioned signs of fracture apply. Vertebral bodies should maintain a rectangular shape. The facets should also be rectangular: height should be greater than width. An asymmetrically shortened facet with prominent joint spaces typically indicates an isolated pillar.

Cartilage and joints

Each intervetebral disc space should be symmetric. Endplates should be parallel. The interfacet joints should be symmetric.

Soft tissues

Displacement or obscuration of the laryngotracheal air column may indicate a haematoma that may be the result of a spinal injury or an injury within the soft tissues of the neck.

Prevertebral soft tissue shadow

Normal characteristics and measurements
- Contour conforms to anterior margin of spine
- Shadow should be <7 mm thick or one third of the thickness of the vertebral body from C2 body to C4
- Shadow should be <21 mm or the thickness of the vertebral body below C4

Causes of thickened prevertebral soft tissue shadow (other than fracture of the cervical spine)

- Haemorrhage from face or fracture of the skull base
- Blood pooling in pharynx
- Prominent lymphoid tissue
- Endotracheal or orogastric tube
- Hypoaeration (child crying)

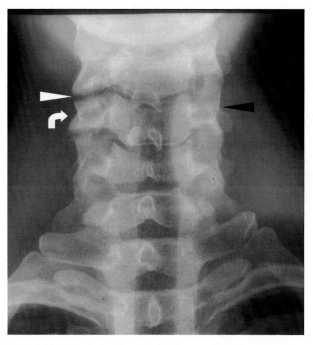

Isolated right C5 articular pillar with foreshortened right facet (curved arrow), and widened adjacent joint space (white arrowhead). Normal left facet (black arrowhead).

Interpretation of open mouth odontoid radiographs

Adequacy

The odontoid process should be visualised clearly, although it is acceptable for the tip to be partially obscured given the rarity of an injury to this site. The C1 and C2 lateral articulations should be discernible. The incisor teeth should not overlap the dens.

Alignment

The margins of the lateral masses of C1 should not overlap the C2 lateral masses. The lateral atlantodental intervals should be within 3 mm from side to side.

A C1 Jefferson burst fracture may be diagnosed when widening of one or both lateral atlantodental spaces with C1 abnormally overriding the lateral masses of C2 laterally is present.

Bones

Follow the contour of the dens and lateral masses. The dens is of primary concern, but all structures merit close inspection.

Cartilage and joints

The C1 and C2 lateral articular surfaces should be parallel, and little or preferably no over-riding should be present.

Soft tissues

Although the soft tissues should be examined, it is unusual for any abnormality to be evident.

Other projections and examination

Computed tomography should be used to evaluate poorly defined or suspicious areas, as well as known fractures. Flexion-extension radiographs and magnetic resonance imaging may be used to evaluate the cervical spine for ligament injury, although the former may be limited in the acute setting. In each case, expert consultation is advocated. If in doubt, scan it.

Pitfalls

All cervical levels from the base of the skull to the T1 superior endplate should be evaluated. If they are not visualised clearly, they cannot be considered adequately evaluated. Particularly troublesome areas include the craniocervical junction to C2 and C7 to T1 – sites prone to injury. Strict attention to the adequacy of the examination is of utmost importance.

At the oropharyngeal level, the soft tissue shadow may be artificially altered or widened by causes other than trauma. Overlapping structures may mimic a fracture. This is most common at the C1 and C2 levels where craniofacial structures may result in such "pseudofractures."

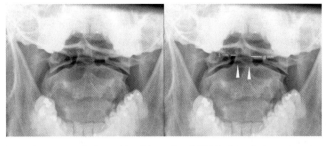

Normal open mouth view with mild rotation (left). The lateral atlantodental intervals (white lines) are within 3 mm (right). Note the overlapping structures (arrowheads) at the odontoid base, which should not be confused with a fracture.

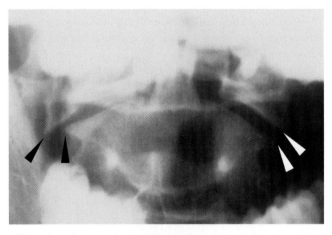

Jefferson burst fracture. Abnormal overlap of the right C1-2 lateral masses (black arrowheads) is seen relative to the left (white arrowheads).

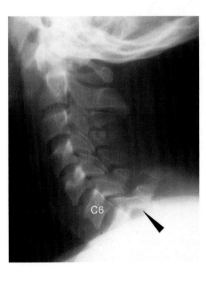

Shoulders obscure C7 and C7-T1 facets rendering the diagnosis of C7-T1 bilateral facet dislocation with bare C7 facets (arrowhead) difficult. Note the C6 and C7 clay shoveler's fractures (same patient illustrated on p. 103).

Congenital variants may cause confusion. In addition, ligamentous laxity in children may cause some confusion, and familiarity with the typical presentations is necessary.

Physiological mimics of injury in children

In children there are normal variants that can confuse or mimic an injury.

- Look for clearly visualised atlanto-occipital joint spaces in infants and young children. Check for a normal posterior axial interval and soft tissue shadow.
- Sometimes more than two thirds of C1 anterior arch above tip of dens (in up to 20% of children younger than eight years).
- Synchondrosis at base of dens may not ossify until the child is 12 years.
- Anterior translation of C2 on C3 and C3 on C4 (occasionally C4 on C5) vertebral bodies can be normal in children up to eight years if normal alignment at the spinolaminar line (pseudosubluxation) is present.
- Congenital variants, such as fusion of C2 and C3 (Klippel-Feil) or hemivertebrae, can cause confusion.

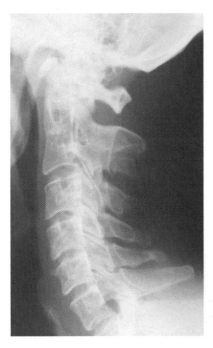

Congenital fusion of C2 and C3 (Klippel-Feil).

Injuries – a summary

- An atlanto-occipital dissociation occurs when the head and neck are separated. It is almost always fatal.
- A Jefferson's burst fracture is an axial compression with a burst fracture of C1 ring
- Odontoid fractures can be classified as three subtypes (types I, II, III), or they can be classified as high or low dens fractures
- A hangman's fracture is a fracture through the pars interarticularis of C2 (spondylolysis of C2)
- Teardrop fractures are usually hyperextension injuries and less commonly hyperflexion injuries
- A unilateral facet dislocation is an anterior dislocation of the vertebral body by less than half of the vertebral body width. On the anteroposterior view there is a sudden change in symmetry seen. The spinous process above the injury is rotated
- A bilateral facet dislocation is an anterior dislocation of the vertebral body by more than half of the width of the vertebral body on the lateral view
- A clay shoveler's fracture is a spinous process fracture of C6 or C7

ABCs systematic assessment

Adequacy
- Check that the the superior endplate of the T1 junction is included on the lateral view
- Check theat the open mouth odontoid view is not rotated

Alignment
- Check the spinal lines (anterior longitudinal ligament line, posterior longitudinal ligament line, spinolaminar ligament line)
- Check laminar space
- Check predental space

Bone
- Check each vertebral body
- Check neural arch

Cartilage and joints
- Check intervertebral disc space
- Check interfacet joints
- Check atlantodental joint and atlanto-occipital joint

Soft tissues
- Check prevertebral soft tissues
- Exclude foreign bodies and teeth
- Check airway and life support devices

CHAPTER 15

Thoracic and Lumbar Spine

Roger N Bodley, Andreas Koureas, Otto Chan

Injuries of the thoracic and lumbar spine tend to occur in falls or road traffic crashes with axial loading, hyperflexion, or extension or distraction forces. Falls are often associated with an element of rotation or shear to the spine. Many conditions predispose to spinal injuries. Suspected abnormalitites are referred to a specialist and more complex imaging, such as computed tomography or magnetic image resonance imaging, will be done. If the plain radiograph is considered normal, however, no further evaluation will be undertaken. This means that medical and medicolegal problems can sometimes occur because of false negative diagnoses.

Clinical examination

Clinical examination of the thoracic and lumbar spine is part of the secondary survey in trauma. It should be deferred until life threatening conditions have been dealt with, and it is done when the patient is "log rolled" (a procedure in which patients are rolled onto their side by a number of staff with minimal movement of the spine). Clinical evaluation can be misleading, especially in patients with distracting injuries. In addition, clinical evaluation is of little value in unconscious patients (who should have a full series of spine films taken irrespective of the clinical findings).

Concentrate on markers that can increase the level of suspicion, and be aware of well recognised associations between trauma in separate locations. Obvious abnormalities can be diagnosed easily. An appreciation of subtle signs is needed for a safe and accurate assessment of the patient, however, so that the threshold of suspicion is raised appropriately.

One of the most important aspects of understanding trauma is appreciating the link between bone and soft tissue injuries. The true nature of an injury (especially a spine injury) is often more apparent if a fracture is thought of as a soft tissue injury in which a bone is also broken and the radiographs are examined with this in mind. A fractured vertebral body is usually of little consequence compared with a damaged spinal cord that may be associated with an apparently minor bone injury or even no readily visible fracture.

In general, the thoracic spine and lumbar spine are better protected than the cervical spine. Large forces are needed to cause serious disruption, and often associated injuries, particularly fractured ribs and solid organ injuries in the abdomen, are present

---

Conditions predisposing to spinal injury

- Degenerative disease
- Malignancy (pathological fracture)
- Osteoporosis, osteopenia, osteomalacia
- Infection
- Paget's disease
- Haemangioma
- Ankylosing spondylitis
- Haemorrhagic disorders
- Developmental or congenital anomalies
- "Hysteria" (must be diagnosed at a senior level)

Thoracolumbar spine injuries – suspect in these situations

Clinical
- Fall from height
- Unconscious patient with multiple injuries
- Paraplegia or neurological symptoms and signs
- Severe local force to the back
- Shock from ruptured spleen or liver
- Haematuria

Radiological
- Fractured sternum (T3-5)
- Fractured ribs posteriorly (adjacent to the fracture)
- Fractured calcaneum (L3-4)
- Fractured scapula

On the other hand, visible soft tissue abnormalities indicate that more serious injury is present, and bone and soft tissue aspects must be analysed. For example, a ruptured liver, spleen, or kidney that is indicated by a fractured rib could kill before more complex imaging to look for spinal stability can be arranged. Stability is a key problem in vertebral injuries, as catastrophic neurological damage may occur in an unstable spine. Predicting stability, however, can be difficult, even with complex modern imaging.

Instability should be assumed until proved otherwise. Appropriate immobilisation, rolling, and turning care should be maintained until an experienced doctor has made a decision to stop. Unstable injuries initially may seem stable because of muscle spasm, but the instability will become apparent when muscle relaxants, analgesia, or anaesthetics are used.

Anatomy

When you assess a radiograph, carefully count each vertebra. Twelve thoracic vertebrae, five lumbar vertebrae, and the sacrum should be present. Variations are common, and it is often difficult to be certain which vertebra is T12 and L1 and which is L4, L5, or S1. This confusion is partly because of the variation in appearance of the 12th rib, but is caused mainly by transitional vertebrae at the lumbosacral junction. The L5 vertebra can be fused partly or completely to the S1 vertebra (sacralisation of L5), or the S1 can be partly or completely separate from S2 vertebra (lumbarisation of S1). Rarely, six lumbar vertebrae may be present. The simplest way to count them is from T1, but the general rule is that the longest and most horizontal transverse process is L3.

The thoracic column is stabilised by strong ligaments (the anterior and posterior longitudinal and interspinous ligaments), the paraspinal muscles, and the ribs that form part of the anterior thoracic cage, although the lower three or four floating ribs have a heavy musculature and provide further support. The lumbar spine has a thick surrounding musculature attached to the transverse processes, which augments the intrinsic stability provided by the discs, ligaments, and facet joints.

Damage tends to occur as the result of a severe direct force or shear or rotational forces such as flexion, extension, or twisting. Stabilisation from the ribs and muscles renders the thoracolumbar junction relatively vulnerable, and most injuries occur between T11 and L2.

In a motor vehicle crash, a seat belt will act as a fulcrum. If the seat belt is a sash belt, the upper and mid-thoracic spine (T3-T5) is often injured by flexion and rotation. The mid lumbar spine can be damaged by flexion if the seat belt is a lap belt.

If the spinal cord is injured, the injuries will be upper motor neurone (hyper-reflexia, spinal shock, and spasticity). The level at which the conus lies varies between T11 and L2, making it vulnerable in thoracolumbar injuries. Below this level, any neurological damage that occurs will be lower motor neurone, because the nerve roots will be damaged.

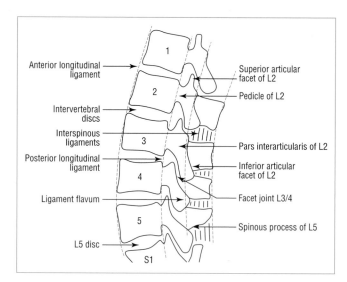

Anatomy of lumbar spine.

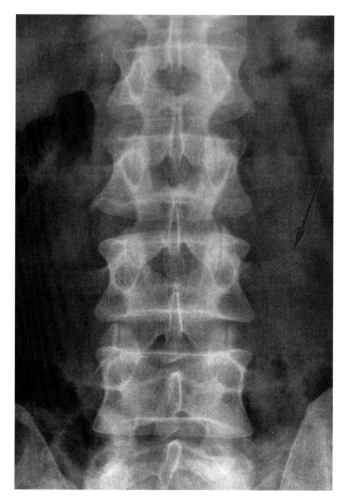

Anteroposterior view of lumbar spine – note length of the transverse process of L3 (arrow).

Abnormalities of the ossification fusion centres may give abnormally shaped vertebrae (hemi or butterfly) or confusing lines that look like fractures (limbus vertebrae).

Underlying disease (such as malignancy, Paget's disease, or osteoporosis) may be found. They should be suspected if the injury seems to be out of proportion to the apparent mechanism and degree of trauma.

ABCs systematic assessment

- **A**dequacy
- **A**lignment
- **B**one
- **C**artilage and joint
- **S**oft tissue

Adequacy

Check that the films are those of the patient. Count the vertebrae and ribs to ensure adequate coverage. The upper thoracic spine can be difficult to show because the shoulders are on the lateral. Patients with major trauma should remain supine until all the radiographical views have been taken and the spine has been assessed and cleared by a specialist.

The routine views are:

- Thoracic spine – anteroposterior and lateral views
- Lumbar spine – anteroposterior and lateral views (coned lumbosacral view is optional)
- Obliques – not routinely indicated in trauma and otherwise rarely indicated except for specific reasons.

It is important that the best possible radiographs are taken in the standard projections. Many potentially confusing lines are present. All clothing, sheets, drip, and electrocardiogram lines should be removed or arranged as smoothly as possible to avoid artefactual lines.

The lateral view should be assessed first to look for gross damage. Often several artefactual lines are present from sheets and pillows. The lateral radiograph should always be examined as if the patient had turned to the right (in keeping with computed tomography and magnetic resonance imaging).

Alignment

On the lateral radiograph, the thoracic spine and lumbar spine have smooth curves that have a gentle midthoracic kyphosis and a slightly more pronounced lumbar lordosis. Check the anterior and posterior longitudinal lines, and the facet lines with no steps or "chicanes."

On the anteroposterior view, the lateral aspect of the vertebral bodies should be aligned, and each side should be checked separately. The pedicles should be oval, clearly distinct, and running in two regular columns, with the spinous processes midway between them. The pedicles gradually separate slightly from L1 to L5. The pedicles on the anteroposterior view, however, should not separate suddenly and be further apart than the pedicle of the vertebrae above and below. Classically, interpedicular widening in trauma is seen in burst fractures.

Mechanisms of thoracic and lumbar spine injury

- Hyperflexion – usually at thoracolumbar junction (T11-L3) with a wedge fracture
- Hyperextension – tears the anterior longitudinal ligament and widens the disc space
- Axial compression – discs and vertebral bodies explode (burst injuries)
- Distraction – rare but may cause ligamentous but no bony injury
- Shearing – slip in any direction, causing disruption of ligaments
- Rotation – leads to facet joint and combination injuries
- Complex or combined vectors

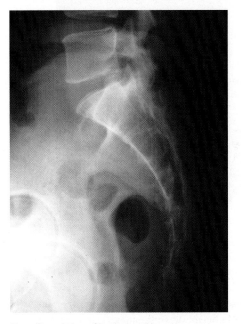

Coned lateral view of lumbosacral junction.

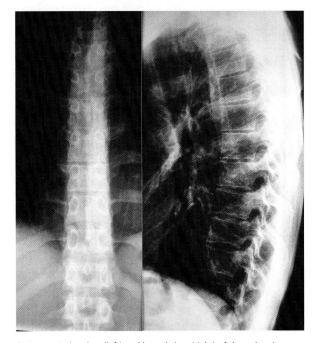

Anteroposterior view (left) and lateral view (right) of thoracic spine.

Bones

Each vertebra should be assessed individually. The bony outlines should be sharp and fine (as in a pen and ink drawing). Imagine trying to draw the contour of each vertebral body and be suspicious of lines that would be best represented by a coarse, ill defined charcoal line. Note breaks in the continuity of the cortex. On the lateral radiograph, a short break in the posterior cortical margin is seen. This is normal. The height of all the vertebral bodies should be similar; loss of height anteriorly indicates a simple wedge or a burst fracture.

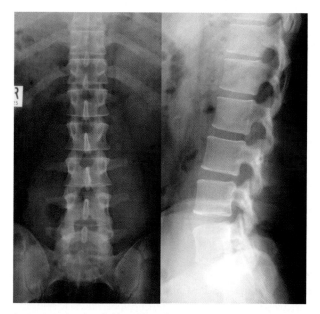

Anteroposterior view (left) and lateral view (right) of lumbar spine.

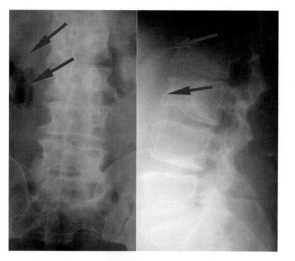

Simple anterior wedge fractures of L1 and L2 (arrows).

Cartilage

Discs and facet joints should have parallel surfaces. Widening, particularly asymmetric, may represent disruption of the joint. The intervertebral disc spaces should be similar and even throughout, with a minimal increase in height down the thoracic and lumbar spine to L4-L5. The L5-S1 disc is usually slightly narrower than the L4/L5 disc. Sudden widening of the intervertebral disc spaces indicates a Chance fracture through the disc. Sudden narrowing is usually degenerative, or occasionally is caused by infection (discitis) or is the result of a crush fracture involving the disc.

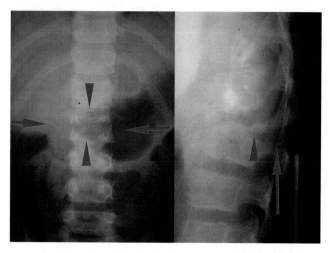

Anteroposterior and lateral view of Chance fracture – note horizontal split in pedicles and transverse processes (arrows) and vertebral body (arrowhead) of L1.

Soft tissues

Soft tissue contours, fat planes, and inter-osseous distances should be smooth and regular. Any focal swelling, haziness, or loss of line should be seen as a possible site of soft tissue damage, and the area should be scrutinised carefully for adjacent bony damage. This is particularly true in the thoracic spine, where the presence of abnormal displaced paraspinal lines in a young patient indicates an injury. Always check the presence and symmetry of psoas shadows. Asymmetric psoas shadows may indicate a retroperitoreal collection (blood or pus).

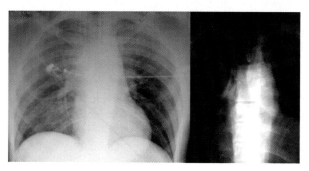

Widened paraspinal lines with fracture of thoracic spine on chest x ray (left) and anteroposterior thoracic spine view (arrows).

Injuries

Two thirds of all injuries occur at T11-L2 and 90% of them between T11-L4. Mid and upper thoracic spine injuries are rare and difficult to see on plain radiographs. In contrast, children have a relatively more mobile spine and injuries are most common at T4/5 and L2. The injuries are often multiple and contiguous.

If an injury mechanism seems too trivial for the observed clinical picture, then there could have been a predisposing cause, making the spine more prone to injury.

Radiological abnormalities of the spine are often seen on a single view only or are better seen on one of two views. The abnormality detected is usually a clue to the underlying injury.

If in doubt, computed tomography is generally the most useful investigation, unless the plain film quality is bad. Repeat radiographs or oblique views are unlikely to help. Magnetic resonance imaging is not usually readily available and the environment in which it is carried out is not trauma friendly.

Injuries invariably are caused by forces that produce extreme movement. They are usually as a result of falls, direct blows, or road traffic accidents. It is important to decide if the injury sustained is stable or unstable. In a stable injury, normal controlled movements will not cause a neurological deficit. Unstable injuries may cause or aggravate neurological damage. Denis's three column model for deciding if an injury is unstable is applicable to the thoracic and lumbar spine. The spine is divided into a posterior, middle, and anterior column. The posterior column includes all of the posterior bony and ligamentous elements. The middle column includes the posterior longitudinal ligament and the elements making up the posterior third of the vertebral body and the intervertebral disc. The anterior column is composed of the remaining portions of the vertebral body and intervertebral disc, and the anterior longitudinal ligament. The spine is stable if the middle column is intact, and the spine is unstable if the middle column is disrupted.

Denis's three column model

- Disruption of two or three columns indicates that an injury is unstable
- Definite disruption of the middle column indicates that an injury is unstable
- Assume instability until it is proved otherwise

Radiological findings for thoracic and lumbar spine injuries

Radiological finding	Injury or point of injury	View finding is best seen on
Widening or narrowing of normal disc space		
Anterior disc margin – anterior longitudinal ligament	Anterior column	Lateral
Posterior disc margin – posterior longitudinal ligament	Middle column	Lateral
Facet joints – disruption	Posterior column	Lateral
Interlaminar line – disruption	Posterior column	Lateral
Widening of soft tissue lines (paraspinal)	Haematoma	Anteroposterior
Distortion in bony margin alignments	Ligamentous disruption	Anteroposterior and lateral
Avulsion fracture from anteroinferior margin	Hyperextension	Lateral
Compression fracture of anterosuperior margin	Hyperflexion	Lateral
Wedging of vertebra	Crush fracture	Lateral
Relative rotation of adjacent vertebral bodies	Unilateral facet dislocation	Lateral
Relative anteroposterior displacement of adjacent bodies	Bilateral facet dislocation	Lateral
Indistinct bony margins and contours	Fracture	Anteroposterior and lateral
Increased interpedicular distance	Burst fracture	Anteroposterior
Poorly visualised pedicles	Comminuted fracture	Anteroposterior
"Apical cap" pleural effusion	Haemothorax	Chest radiograph

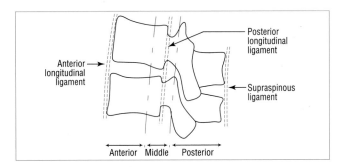

Denis's three column model is used to decide if an injury is unstable.

Injuries – a summary

- A wedge fracture is an isolated anterior body compression fracture
- A stable burst fracture is rare. The anterior and middle columns are compressed, but the posterior column is still intact
- An unstable burst fracture is common. It is a fracture of the sagittal body, and there is widening of the pedicles and disruption of the bony ring
- A Chance fracture is common. It is a hyperflexion (lap belt) injury with a horizontal body fracture with distraction, extending into the pedicles and posterior elements. Rarely, distraction is through the disc
- A translation injury is unstable. Alignment is disrupted by a shear injury in all three planes
- An unstable flexion or distraction occurs when the anterior column is compressed with extension of the middle column and posterior column. It is usually unstable

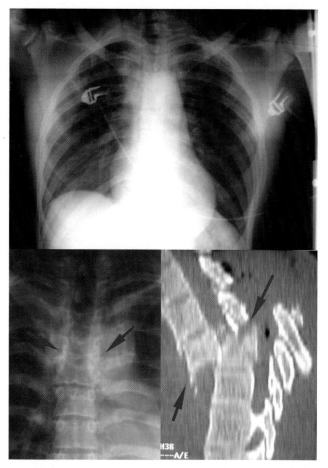

Translation injury on T5 and T6. Chest radiograph (top), anteroposterior view of thoracic spine (bottom left) and sagittal reconstruction computed tomography of thoracic spine showing fracture dislocation T5 and T6 (arrows).

ABCs systematic assessment

Alignment
- Check smooth contours on lateral view
- Check spinal lines (anterior longitudinal ligament line, posterior longitudinal ligament line, spinolaminar ligament line, and supra-spinous ligament line) on lateral view
- Check lateral margins of vertebral body on anteroposterior view for fractures or displacment

Bones
- Check each vertebra separately for fractures
- Make sure anterior, middle, and posterior columns are intact

Cartilage
- Check for widening or narrowing of intervertebral disc spaces
- Check facets and interspinous distances

Soft tissues
- Check for abnormal soft tissues

KEY POINTS

- Most injuries are caused by severe forces
- Most injuries are near the thoracolumbar region
- Injuries in the upper and mid-thoracic spine are rare in adults
- Spinal injuries are often associated with injuries elsewhere
- Use a systematic approach to avoid missing subtle yet serious injuries

CHAPTER 16

Emergency Paediatric Radiology

Marina J Easty, Rosy Jalan

Children make up about one third of all patients who attend emergency departments. Skeletal injuries in infants (<1 year), children (>1 year), adolescents, and adults all differ greatly.

Children are more agile, more flexible, and lighter than adults. When they fall, the forces generated are smaller. Boys sustain more injuries than girls, and most injuries occur at home or playing sport at school.

Fractures in infants are rare. Toddlers tend to sustain skull and tibial fractures, whereas distal forearm, ankle, and foot injuries are often seen in schoolchildren.

Emergency paediatrics

- Children often present at accident and emergency departments
- Boys present more commonly than girls
- Seasonal variations in the type of injury occur
- Children have different problems to adults

Definitions used in paediatric medicine

- Premature infant: ≤ 37 weeks' gestation
- Neonate: birth to 28 days old
- Infant: 1 month to 1 year old
- Toddler: 1-3 years old
- Child: ≥ 3 years old

This chapter gives an overview of common paediatric fractures and other radiological emergencies. It explains a systematic approach on how to interpret the relevant radiographs, but conditions are not dealt with in detail. Common fractures in the paediatric population will be discussed, followed by a list of common abdominal and other childhood emergencies.

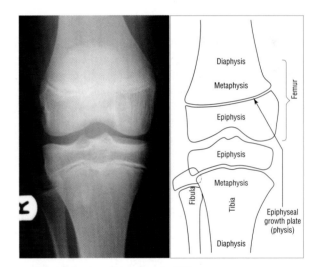

Anteroposterior view of right knee in child.

Fractures

Fractures in children are different to those in adults because of anatomical, biomechanical, and physiological differences. In addition, a range of fractures is caused in children, because paediatric bones are softer and more pliable than adult bones.

Anatomy

At birth, many bones or the ends of bones are not visible. In time, ossification centres appear (sometimes several), then they enlarge and coalesce, eventually fusing to the adjacent bone. The time interval between these changes varies from bone to bone, but predictable timescales vary slightly between boys and girls, and between different ethnic origins.

The physis (growth plate) is avascular after infancy. Damage to this area is shown radiographically by changes in its width or changes in adjacent bone. Damage to the epiphyseal vessels leads to death of the physeal chondrocytes and growth arrest.

The periosteum in the paediatric population is thick and strong and can produce exuberant callus. The attachment of the periosteum to the shaft of the bone is loose in children, and so periosteal reactions and subperiosteal collections are common.

Biomechanical differences

Paediatric bones are more porous than adult bones, and they can bend more without breaking. The weak point lies at the physis, and so physeal fractures are common before bony fusion. The thick, strong periosteum resists displacement of the fracture (unless it is torn).

Physiological differences

Fractures heal faster in children than in adults, and remodelling is quicker because children have rapid bone turnover. Normal alignment occurs in the plane of motion of the adjacent joint. Fracture healing results in longitudinal overgrowth, therefore in long bone diaphyseal fractures overlap (up to 2 cm of bone) is accepted. The fracture should be described like an adult fracture – for example, transverse, oblique, comminuted, or compound. After the age of 12 years, fractures are treated more like those in the adult population due to slower remodelling.

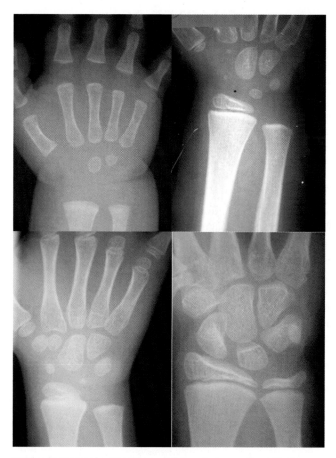

Serial radiographs of wrist with no epiphyses at one year (top left), three years (top right), six years (bottom left), and 12 years (bottom right).

Types of fracture

Complete diaphyseal fractures – The fracture site should be examined for an underlying bony abnormality, such as a bone cyst or generalised demineralisation. For infants and the non-ambulant a careful history should be taken to exclude non-accidental injury.

Torus or buckle fractures – failure on the compression side of a bending bone causes a torus or buckle fracture – an outward buckling of the cortex margin (*torus* is a latin term for bulge or swelling). Torus fractures usually occur near the metaphysis, where the cortex is thinnest. They often occur at the distal radius due to a fall on an outstretched hand.

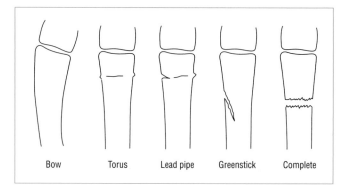

Bow   Torus   Lead pipe   Greenstick   Complete

Types of fracture.

Greenstick fracture – When a bone is bent beyond its limits, a greenstick fracture is produced. It is caused by the bone bending on the compression side, with complete failure on the tension side of the bone. The fracture may later hinge open because of muscle pull.

Bowing fractures – caused by acute plastic deformation of the bone secondary to longitudinal stress. An increase in longitudinal compression leads to bowing, buckle fractures, lead pipe fractures, greenstick fractures, and complete fractures.

Physeal fractures

Salter-Harris classification

The standard classification for physeal injuries is that of Salter and Harris. This classification divides the common types (I-IV) according to the course of the fracture through the physis and the adjacent epiphyseal and metaphyseal bone. Type V injuries are rare, may be occult radiographically, and are caused by compression of the physeal cartilage. Several additions have been made to the original classification, although they will not be discussed in this chapter.

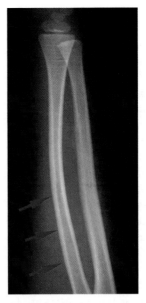
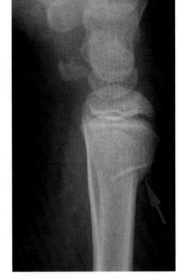

Midshaft fracture of ulna and a bow fracture of the radius (arrow).

Lead pipe fracture (arrow).

Salter-Harris classification

- Type I – **S**lipped or **s**eparated
- Type II – **A**bove
- Type II – **L**ower
- Type IV – **T**hrough
- Type V – **E**venly **r**ammed

Common sites of physeal injuries

Type I (incidence 6% of Salter-Harris fractures)
- Common locations – proximal humerus, distal humerus, proximal femur, distal tibia, and distal fibula

Type II (incidence 75% of Salter-Harris fractures)
- Common locations – distal radius, distal tibia, distal fibula, distal femur, distal ulna, and phalanges

Type III (incidence 8% of Salter-Harris fractures)
- Common locations – distal tibia, proximal tibia, and distal femur

Type IV (incidence 10% of Salter-Harris fractures)
- Common locations – distal humerus, and distal tibia

Type V (incidence 1% of Salter-Harris fractures)
- Common locations – ankle and knee

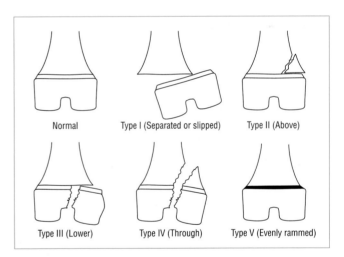

Salter-Harris classification for physical injuries.

Type I

These are caused by a shearing stress through the physis. Most apophyseal injuries and slipped upper femoral epiphyses are type I fractures. Neonates may sustain these fractures at the proximal humerus. In the prepubertal child, a supination-inversion injury of the ankle may result in a type I fracture through the distal fibula. Invariably, this fracture will be reduced at the time of presentation and radiographical assessment. Type I fractures have a good prognosis.

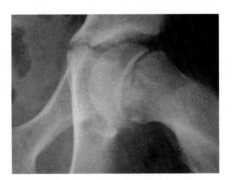

Salter-Harris type I fracture – slipped upper femoral epiphysis of the left hip.

Type II

These are the most common physeal fractures (75% of physeal fractures). The avulsion or shearing force fractures the physis and extends into the metaphysis. Radiographs show a triangular metaphyseal fracture known as the Thurston-Holland fragment. Between one third and one half of all type II injuries involve the distal radius. Reduction of the fracture is usually uncomplicated, and these injuries have a good prognosis.

Type III

Type III injuries are partly intra-articular, with splitting of the epiphysis and a transverse fracture through the physis. As they involve all layers of the physis, they cause growth arrest. Type III injuries occur in adolescents about the time of closure of the physis, and they often require operative reduction to prevent displacement.

Type IV

These injuries cross the epiphysis, physis, and metaphysis. They are caused by a longitudinally orientated splitting force, and they usually arise in the distal humerus or distal tibia. These injuries generally require open reduction to oppose the fracture fragments. Consequent angulation and leg length abnormalities may occur.

Type V

Type V injuries are often diagnosed in retrospect, when growth arrest occurs after the injury. They are caused by a substantial loading or compressive force that damages the vascular supply and germinal cells of the growth plate. Most isolated type V injuries occur in the ankle or knee.

Elbow injuries

Injuries of the three bones around the elbow are the most common fractures seen in infancy and childhood. There are six secondary ossification centres around the elbow (CRITOL, or CRITOE).

The age of the appearance of ossification centres is variable. The ossification centres of the distal humerus fuse with each other and then with the distal humerus in adolescents aged between 14 and 16 years. The medial or internal epicondyle may not fuse until a young person is 19 years of age.

The fat pads (anterior and posterior) around the elbow are elevated when a joint effusion is present. This may be seen with trauma, but it is also seen with haemorrhage, infection, inflammation, and malignancy.

Traumatic joint effusions are caused by a dislocation or fracture of the humerus, radius, or ulna. More than 90% of children with an elevated posterior fat pad sign have a fracture. The radial head fracture is the most frequent occult injury, but "pulled elbows" (dislocated radial head epiphysis which has relocated at the time of imaging), supracondylar fractures, and lateral condylar fractures may all be difficult to see.

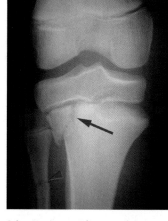

Salter-Harris type II fracture of the proximal tibia. Note the transverse fracture of proximal fibula (arrowhead).

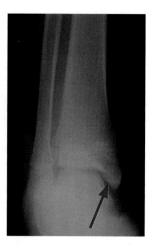

Salter-Harris type III fracture of distal tibial epiphyses (arrow).

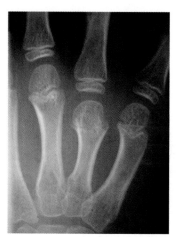

Salter-Harris type V fracture of fourth metacarpal. A load bearing force leads to a compression fracture.

Average age of appearance of ossification centres (CRITOL)*

- **C**apitellum – 12 months
- **R**adial head – 3-6 years
- **I**nternal epicondyle – 4-7 years
- **T**rochlear – 7-10 years
- **O**lecranon – 6-10 years
- **L**ateral or **e**xternal epicondyle – 11-14 years

*Appear earlier in girls

Interpretation of the elbow radiograph

Four sets of lines help interpretation.

Anterior humeral line – normally passes through the middle third of the ossified capitellum. With a supracondylar fracture, and dorsal angulation of the distal humeral fragment, this line passes in front of the anterior third of the capitellum.

Radiocapitellar line – this line is drawn through the centre of the radial shaft and passes through the capitellum on all radiographic views. This line confirms articulation between the radial head and capitellum. If the line does not pass through the capitellum, dislocation of the radial head is likely.

Coronoid line – this is the concave line drawn along the coronoid fossa. An extension of this line touches or projects slightly anterior to the capitellum and helps to show displacement of the capitellum in supracondylar fractures.

X sign (hour glass) – the X is made up of the olecranon and coronoid fossa on the lateral view: disruption indicates a supracondylar fracture.

Supracondylar fractures

These are the most common fractures of the elbow in children aged 5-10 years. These fractures are hyperextension injuries, and are usually caused by a fall onto an outstretched hand.

On a lateral radiograph of the elbow, a positive posterior fat pad sign is seen, the X sign is disrupted, and the anterior humeral line passes through or anterior to the anterior third of the capitellum. The fracture line may be easier to identify on the lateral view.

Lateral condylar fractures

This is the second most common fracture of the elbow in children aged 2-8 years. This injury is caused by hyperextension with varus stress. This fracture is usually a Salter-Harris type IV injury that involves a small fragment of metaphysis extending into the unossified epiphysis of the lateral humeral condyle.

Medial epicondyle fractures

About 10% of elbow injuries are fractures of the medial epicondyle. They occur in children aged 8-15 years.

The fracture is caused by hyperextension with valgus stress. The medial epicondyle is the site of attachment of the forearm flexor muscles and the ulnar collateral ligament. The insertion is vulnerable to valgus stress and to excessive muscle pull (usually during throwing).

The radiograph will usually show soft tissue swelling overlying the medial epicondyle. Care must be taken in children younger than five years because the epicondyle will not have ossified. Injuries range from separation of the epicondyle to dislocation and intra-articular entrapment of the epicondyle. The epicondyle will not be in its usual position. Medial epicondyle fractures are caused by rotation applied to the forearm bones causing avulsion of the epicondyle by the flexor pronator tendon.

Radial head fractures

About 9% of elbow injuries in children of 6-13 years are radial head fractures. They are caused by a valgus force applied to the bones below the elbow leading to an impaction fracture.

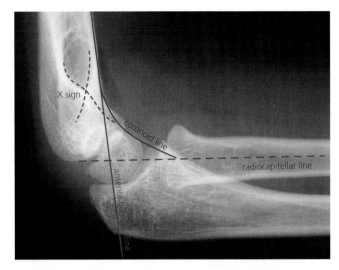

Lines on elbow radiograph (anterior humeral line, radiocapitellar line, coronoid line, X sign).

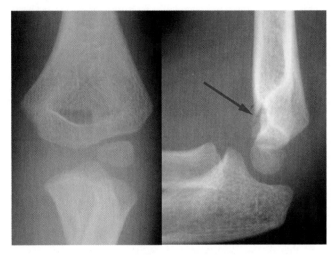

Supracondylar fracture. Note how subtle the fracture line can be on the anteroposterior view (left). The lateral view on the right shows a positive anterior humeral line and disruption of the X (positive X sign) (arrow).

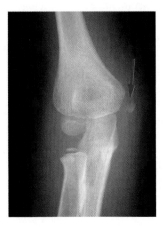

Fracture dislocation of the medial epicondyle (arrow).

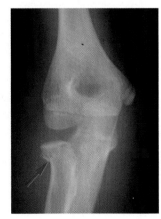

Fracture of the radial neck (arrow).

The most common radial head fracture is a Salter-Harris type II injury. Buckle fractures may be subtle. The fracture is often difficult to detect, however, elevated fat pads are often seen on radiographs.

Pulled elbow

This injury is common in infants and young children younger than three years. It is caused by a sharp pull on the arm or lifting the child by one arm. It is extremely painful, and the child will refuse to move the arm. There is a subluxation of the radial head from the annular ligament, with partial tearing of the ligament and entrapment of a portion of the ligament in the joint space.

Radiographs normally are unhelpful, although positioning the child for the lateral radiograph may lead to reduction of the subluxation.

Forearm fractures

These include Monteggia fractures and Galeazzi fractures. A Monteggia fracture is a fracture of the proximal to the middle third of the shaft of the ulna with a dislocated radial head. Care must be taken when assessing apparent isolated ulna fractures, so that a radial head dislocation is excluded. Galeazzi fractures are rare in children. The radius is fractured and dislocation of the distal radio-ulnar joint is present.

Painful hips

Perthes disease (Legg-Calve-Perthes disease) occurs commonly in Caucasian boys. A boy to girl ratio of 4:1 is seen. Bilateral disease is present in up to 13% of patients who present with Perthes disease. The age of presentation ranges from 3-12 years, with children typically presenting at 5-8 years. Girls present at a younger age. Children with Perthes disease invariably have delayed bone age. They have pain in the hip, groin, thigh, or knee, and they have limited internal rotation.

Perthes disease is idiopathic avascular necrosis of the femoral capital epiphysis. The disease sometimes occurs after trauma or an effusion. The cause of Perthes disease, however, is not known.

The typical radiological findings depend on the stage of the disease. Early findings may show a small femoral capital epiphysis with a subchondral lucency. Magnetic resonance imaging and scintigraphy of the hip may pick up early changes better than plain radiography. Marrow oedema may be seen on a magnetic resonance image and absent radionuclide uptake in the affected epiphysis in the bone scan. Findings on plain radiography that occur later are fragmentation, flattening, and sclerosis of the femoral capital epiphysis. Coxa magna may also develop during the reparative stage. Treatment may be minimal or simply rest. The aim is to prevent the hip subluxing, prevent pain, and minimise degenerative disease.

Slipped upper femoral epiphysis

The boy to girl ratio is 2.5:1. The age of presentation is 12-15 years in boys and 10-13 years in girls. There may be familial cases of slipped upper femoral epiphysis.

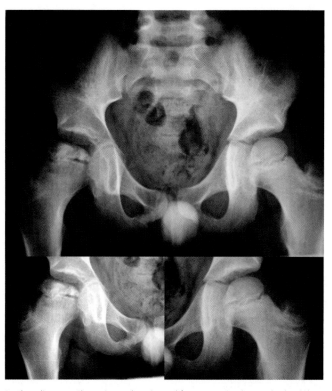

Perthes disease – Flattening, sclerosis, and fragmentation is seen in the right femoral capital epiphysis (arrow) compared with the normal left epiphysis of a 7 year old boy.

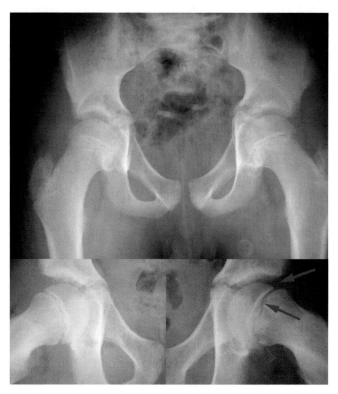

Slipped upper femoral epiphysis – anteroposterior view shows subtle changes but the frog's leg lateral of the left hip shows subtle widening of the physis (arrow). The inferior margin is blurred and the epiphysis has slipped inferomedially (arrowhead) compared with the right hip.

Children with slipped upper femoral epiphysis are usually overweight or tall for their age and have some delay in skeletal maturation. Half of affected patients give a history of serious trauma. The most common presentation is hip pain and limp, but 25% of patients complain of knee pain. Bilateral slip occurs in 20-32% of patients, and more commonly in girls.

Slipped upper femoral epiphysis is a Salter-Harris type I injury. The initial imaging is an anteroposterioir pelvic radiograph and a frog's leg lateral view of both hips.

The imaging findings may be subtle on the anteroposterior projection. The slip is initially posterior and therefore the frog's leg lateral view is essential, as only 75% of patients have a significant medial component to the slip.

The frontal view shows osteopenia of the affected femur. The physis may be wide. The metaphyseal margin of the physis is usually blurred. A line drawn tangential to the lateral femoral neck should bisect the femoral capital epiphysis, so that about one sixth of the diameter of the femoral capital epiphysis is lateral to this line. The epiphyseal height is reduced because of the posterior slip. In chronic slip, callus formation may be seen.

Treatment is to fix the hip to prevent further slip. The hip is pinned in situ, because realignment may lead to avascular necrosis.

Septic arthritis

Fever, pain, a raised white cell count, and raised levels of acute phase proteins may increase suspicion of septic arthritis. An ultrasound scan of the hip follows the plain imaging. The findings on the plain film may be subtle and include osteopenia of the femur and bowing of the gluteus fat pad. The femoral head may be displaced laterally, with widening of the medial joint space caused by accumulated fluid. The hip joint is then imaged in the sagittal plane by ultrasonography, with comparison views of the unaffected side. Pus in the joint will cause bowing of the capsule, and debris may be seen in the fluid. Orthopaedic surgeons treat the patient by washing out the hip joint.

Avulsion fractures around the hips

Avulsion fractures around the pelvic bones are common in children. Common sites are the anterior superior iliac spine (ASIS), the anterior inferior iliac spine (AIIS), and the ischial tuberosity. Plain films, and careful clinical examination, will usually identify these injuries.

Non-accidental injury

The hallmark of this condition is clinical and radiographical evidence of repeated injury. It was first described by Caffey in 1946, although, in fact, Tardieu reported these injuries in infants in the French literature in 1860.

Skeletal presentations of non-accidental injury tend to occur in children who cannot talk, hence 50% occur before the age of one year and 80% by the age of two years. In 50% of proved cases of non-accidental injury, the skeletal survey is normal.

Injuries with a delayed presentation, an unlikely explanation, a changing history, an unusual mechanism, or multiple fractures of differing ages should raise the suspicion of non-accidental injury. The importance of taking an accurate history in these cases cannot

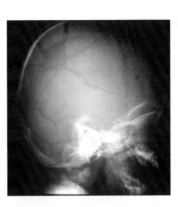

Complex skull fracture in nonaccidental injury.

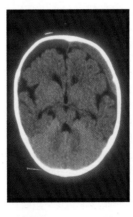

Bilateral subdural haematomas of different ages in a 6 month old baby with implausible history from parents.

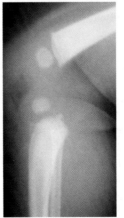

Metaphyseal corner fracture seen in the proximal tibia.

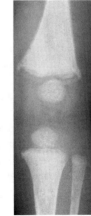

Metaphyseal bucket handle fracture of the distal femur and a subtle bucket handle of the proximal tibia.

be overstated. The height of the fall, mechanism of the fall, the leading part involved, and the surface onto which the child fell all need to be ascertained, as does the exact timing of the injury. Remember that a fall from a bed onto a carpeted floor usually will not lead to a fracture in a child with normal bones. Retinal haemorrhages caused by shaking are an important sign in non-accidental injury, as are marks on the skin, such as bruises and burns.

Many battered children present with skull fractures and underlying subdural haematomas. An unexplained skull fracture, particularly one that crosses sutures, or a diastased fracture are suggestive of non-accidental injury. A computed tomography scan of the brain will show intracerebral injuries.

The classic fractures in non-accidental injury are metaphyseal corner fractures, caused by violent shaking or twisting of the baby; however, less than 50% of babies present with metaphyseal fractures. They may present with other injuries, such as spiral or oblique fractures of the long bones, soft tissue injuries, or abdominal injuries (pancreatic and duodenal injuries). In babies younger than one year, an isolated long bone fracture should be considered suggestive of non-accidental injury, and a skeletal survey may be warranted.

Rib, clavicular, spine, pelvis, and scapular fractures may all be seen in non-accidental injury. Rib fractures, particularly posterior fractures, are highly suggestive of non-accidental injury, although lateral and anterior fractures are common in non-accidental injury. They result from squeezing the child. Anterior fractures occur by squeezing and shaking the child and are caused by costochondral separation. The fractures are seen best when callus forms, so a repeat chest radiograph is advised 10 days after presentation.

Chest emergencies

Inhaled foreign body

An expiratory radiograph is advised to reveal air trapping. The chest radiograph may show an area of consolidation, collapse, or air trapping, with a transradiant lung. The foreign body may be visible.

Other chest emergencies

Asthma – No radiological abnormality is seen, except a degree of air trapping with large volume lungs. It is important to exclude a pneumothorax.

Pneumonia – May present as a focal area of consolidation (**air-space shadowing**).

Pleural empyema – An ultrasound scan will show the pleural effusion and the presence of loculations. Drainage guided by ultrasonography is advocated.

Pneumothorax – May be difficult to diagnose if the chest radiograph has been taken supine.

Cardiac abnormalities – Chest radiograph may show cardiac enlargement, a right sided aortic arch, elevation of the cardiac apex, or selective chamber enlargement, but it is often unhelpful. Referral to specialists (particularly for echocardiography) is advised for further management.

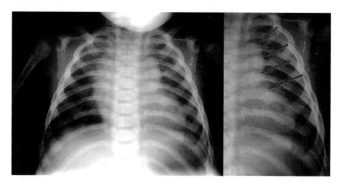

Multiple rib fractures. Chest radiographs and anteroposterior magnified view showing multiple rib fractures.

Skeletal survey for non-accidental injury

- Skull radiograph – anteroposterior and lateral views, and Townes if an occipital fracture is suspected
- Lateral view of the whole spine
- Chest radiograph – repeat in 10 days
- Oblique views of the ribs
- Anteroposterior view of abdomen and pelvis
- Frontal views of arms and hands
- Frontal views of legs and feet
- Computed tomography scan of the brain

Note that lateral views of fractured bones are also advised

If the patient has a history of an inhaled foreign body, the chest film may be normal and a bronchoscopy may be required

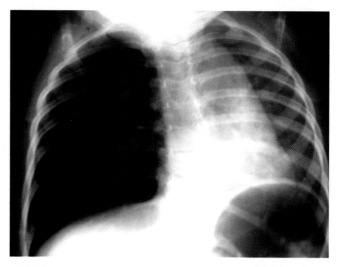

Inhaled foreign body on chest radiograph with hyperinflated and transradiant right lung.

Acute abdominal emergencies

Clinical examination and ultrasonography are the initial investigations for children with acute abdominal emergencies. Unlike adults, computed tomography should be reserved for specific conditions in children and only requested by the paediatric specialists. A list of possible conditions is given in the box, without detailed description of the radiological abnormalities. Plain abdominal radiographs may be helpful in neonates but are less useful in older children.

Renal tract emergencies

If renal abnormalities are suspected, request an ultrasound scan.

Renal masses
- Hydronephrosis
- Complicated duplex kidney
- Multicystic dysplastic kidney
- Renal tumour – usually a Wilms' tumour in children younger than 10 years with mesoblastic nephroma diagnosed at birth
- Autosomal recessive polycystic kidney disease

Renal abnormalities
- Urinary tract infection
- Renal stones
- Haematuria, trauma, infection, renal vein thrombosis, glomerulonephritis, and nephrotic syndrome

Further reading

Borden S. Roentgen recognition of acute plastic bowing of the forearm in children. *AJR* 1975;**125**:524-30

Rang M. *Children's fractures*. Philadelphia: JP Lippincott, 1983

Salter RB, Harris WB. Injuries involving the epiphyseal plate. *J Bone Joint Surg Am* 1963;**45**:587-622

Acute abdominal emergencies

Obstruction in the neonate
High obstruction
- Malrotation and volvulus
- Duodenal atresia, duodenal web, duodenal stenosis, and annular pancreas all give a "double bubble" appearance
- Jejunal atresia
- Duodenal duplication cyst causing obstruction

Low obstruction
- Hirschsprung's disease
- Meconium ileus. May be diagnosed in utero. Note meconium peritonitis with calcification
- Meconium plug syndrome (left sided microcolon)
- Ileal atresia
- Ano-rectal malformation
- Anal stenosis
- Milk curd obstruction
- Obstructed hernia

Obstruction in infants and older children
- Intussusception, diagnosed with ultrasonography
- Appendicitis
- Adhesion obstruction
- Hernia
- Constipation
- Do not forget malrotation at all ages

Abdominal masses
- Duplication cysts
- Ovarian cysts
- Mesenteric cysts
- Tumours

CHAPTER 17

Major Trauma

Otto Chan, Alastair Wilson, Michael Walsh

Advanced trauma life support is the standard method for the initial management of severely injured patients. The principle is simple – treat the greatest threat to life first. Loss of airway will kill before inability to breathe, and inability to breathe will kill before bleeding and loss of circulation. A definitive diagnosis is not necessary to treat the patient initially. The most important point to remember is that no harm should be done to the patient during treatment. The management of severely injured patients is divided into the primary and secondary survey. This article deals with the imaging during the primary survey.

Primary survey

The primary survey comprises a rapid evaluation of the patient, resuscitation, and institution of life preserving treatment. This process is called the ABCDE of trauma. Adjuncts to the primary survey include relevant imaging during resuscitation and re-evaluation.

In practice, most of the steps of the ABCDE are carried out simultaneously by a trauma team. Anaesthetists will usually deal with the airway and intravenous access while the surgeon evaluates the chest, abdomen, and pelvis for potential life threatening injuries.

Imaging is requested as part of the primary survey while the patient is assessed, life threatening injuries are dealt with, and resuscitation procedures instituted. Imaging should not be performed if it interferes with the rest of the primary survey or definitive care, and only investigations that may have a direct effect on the patient's initial problems should be done.

Examples of imaging done as part of the primary survey include radiographs of the supine anteroposterior chest, supine pelvis, and lateral cervical spine (although this can be delayed if necessary); and limited ultrasonography (also known as FAST, focused assessment with sonography for trauma).

ABCDE of trauma

- **A**irway and cervical spine control
- **B**reathing and ventilation
- **C**irculation and haemorrhage control
- **D**isability and neurological status
- **E**xposure and environment

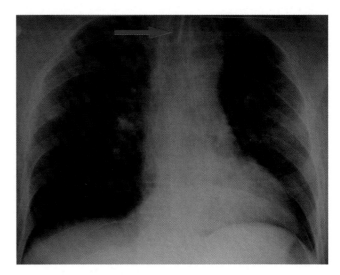

Supine radiograph showing endotracheal tube 5 cm above carina (arrow).

Airway and cervical spine control

The airway should be assessed for patency. Foreign bodies and vomit should be removed and facial, mandibular, tracheal, and laryngeal injuries should be excluded clinically.

If the patient is conscious and talking, there is usually no immediate need for airway intervention. If the patient is unconscious and breathing spontaneously, an oropharyngeal airway may suffice as a temporary measure. Any patient who has a head injury and a score on the Glasgow coma scale of 8 or less should be intubated. However, intubation may be required for optimal control of airways in patients with higher scores.

If the patient has been intubated, a chest radiograph should be taken to check the position of the endotracheal tube. The tip of the tube should not lie below the level of the aortic arch in a supine chest radiograph and a minimum of 3.5 cm (and preferably 5 cm) above the carina.

Care should be taken to avoid worsening a potential cervical spine injury while establishing and safeguarding an airway. If the airway has been secured and the neck immobilised the cervical spine radiograph can be delayed. The cervical spine should be immobilised with a cervical collar, sandbag, and tape. Should the collar need to be removed, an experienced member of the trauma team should carry out in-line manual immobilisation of the head and neck.

Breathing and ventilation

A patent airway does not guarantee adequate ventilation. The lungs, chest wall, and diaphragm must be assessed for potential injuries that could compromise ventilation acutely. These injuries include tension pneumothorax, tension haemothorax, flail chest, and open pneumothorax. It can be difficult to exclude these injuries in a patient with multiple trauma. A chest radiograph must be taken as soon as possible. If the patient is subsequently intubated or ventilated, a second radiograph should be taken to confirm that the endotracheal tube is in a satisfactory position and that life threatening injuries have not been made worse. Ventilation can cause a simple pneumothorax to become a tension pneumothorax.

Circulation and haemorrhage control

The patient's haemodynamic state must be assessed quickly and accurately because bleeding is a major cause of preventable death. Clinical evaluation is essential, in particular, the level of consciousness, skin colour, and pulse. Any external source of bleeding should be identified and dealt with immediately using manual pressure. When the examination or history suggests internal injury, a pelvic radiograph should be taken and limited ultrasonography (FAST) done to exclude hidden blood loss. The presence of a pelvic fracture or free fluid on ultrasonography mandates a specialist opinion.

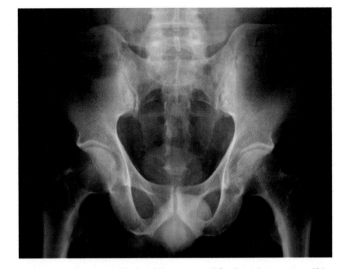

Radiograph of supine pelvis should be requested for the primary survey. This radiograph shows no abnormality.

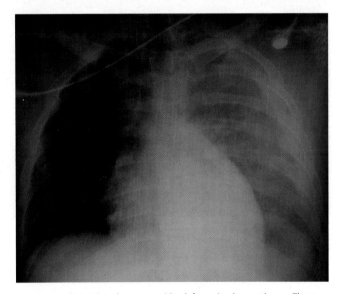

Anteroposterior supine chest x ray with a left tension haemothorax. There is an opaque left haemothorax with evidence of contralateral shift of the mediastinum.

Main causes of hidden blood loss

- Chest, abdomen, and retroperitoneal injuries
- Pelvic fractures
- Multiple long bone fractures

Disability (neurological examination)

The patient's neurological state is assessed with the Glasgow coma scale. It is easy and quick to use and is a determinant of patient outcome and possible further management.

FAST can be performed by a physician, surgeon, or radiologist and has been shown to be valuable in the assessment of blunt trauma patients in the emergency room, especially in unstable patients with multiple injuries. Ultrasonography should be performed in five areas. These areas are the 5 Ps – perihepatic, peripluric, and pelvis in the abdomen, and pericardial (to exclude a pericardial tamponade) and pleural (to detect fluid or a pneumothorax) in the chest or consolidated lung.

All patients with a head injury should have computed tomography of the head, especially if they have lost consciousness, have amnesia, or severe headaches. Up to 18% of patients with mild head injuries have abnormalities on computed tomography, and 5% of these patients may require surgery.

Glasgow coma scale score

Eye opening (graded 1-4)
- Spontaneous – 4
- To speech – 3
- To pain – 2
- None – 1

Verbal response (graded 1-5)
- Orientated – 5
- Confused conversation – 4
- Inappropriate words – 3
- Incomprehensible sounds – 2
- None – 1

Best motor response (graded 1-6)
- Obeys command – 6
- Localises pain – 5
- Normal flexion – 4
- Abnormal flexion – 3
- Extension (decerebrate) – 2
- None – 1

Maximum score 15, minimum score 3
Mild injury 14-15
Moderate injury 9-13
Severe injury 3-8
Coma ≤8

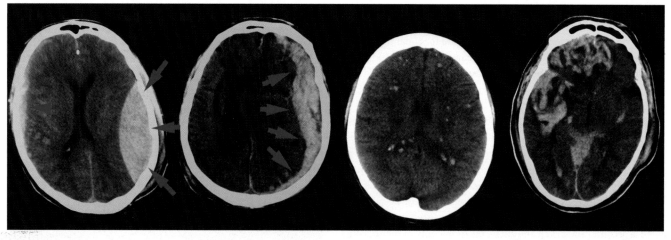

Left extradural haematoma (arrows) and a subtle right subdural (arrowhead) haematoma (far left), large subdural haematoma (arrows) (middle left), diffuse axonal injury (middle right) and combination injuries (right).

> **If the patient has a head, scan it – missing a serious head injury may have catastrophic consequences**

Computed tomography should be done as soon as possible because morbidity and mortality rises substantially if surgery is delayed. The intracranial findings of computed tomography may include no abnormality, extradural haematoma, subdural haematoma, contusions and intracerebral haematomas, subarachnoid blood, diffuse axonal injury, and combination injuries.

The National Institute of Clinical Excellence (NICE) introduced UK guidelines for management of head injury in 2003 that support the advanced trauma life support guidelines. They emphasise that computed tomography must be done within an hour of the patient arriving at the hospital.

Exposure and environment

The patient should be fully exposed (by cutting off all clothes) to allow a full examination. It is, however, critical to keep the patient

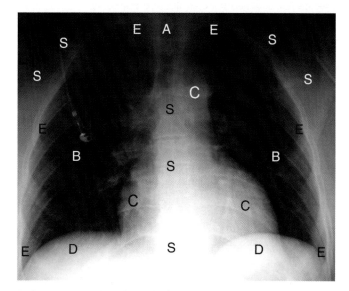

Supine anteroposterior radiograph of normal chest with ABCDEs interpretation.

warm with blankets and a heated emergency room. Large volumes of fluids may be infused, and these intravenous fluids should be warmed.

Adjuncts to primary survey and resuscitation

As a minimum, patients should have electrocardiography, their blood pressure monitored, pulse oximetry, a nasogastric tube, and a urinary catheter. Blood gases should also be monitored. If a fracture at the base of the skull is suspected, the nasogastric tube can be inserted after computed tomography of the head or an orogastric tube placed.

Interpreting primary survey images

All imaging must be supervised and done without fuss or undue delay and with meticulous technique. Attention to detail is essential. In particular, the film must be labelled (including the patient's name and a side marker).

The supine chest radiograph should be taken as soon as possible after the patient has been exposed and centred correctly. Attention must be paid to stop patients being rotated and keeping them in the middle of the trolley.

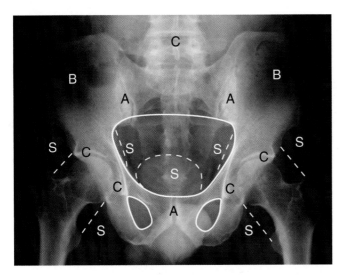

Radiograph of supine pelvis showing ABCDEs interpretation.

ABCDEs interpretation of the supine chest radiograph

Airways
- Check trachea is clear and central
- Is airway patent?
- Check position of endotracheal tube
- Are there any teeth or foreign bodies?
- Check all lines and tubes

Breathing
- Exclude tension pneumothorax and haemothorax
- Check there is no radiological flail segment
- Exclude rib fractures
- Check lungs are clear

Circulation
- Check heart size and mediastinal contours are normal
- Make sure that the aortic arch is clearly seen
- Check the hila and vascular markings are normal

Diaphragm
- Check that diaphragms appear normal (size, shape, and position)
- Can both diaphragms be clearly seen?
- Check under each diaphragm

Edges
- Check the pleura and costophrenic recesses
- Exclude a subtle pneumothorax or effusion

Soft tissues and skeleton
- Look for surgical emphysema
- Check clavicles and shoulders and exclude rib fractures
- Look at the paraspinal lines and check the spine

ABCs interpretation of pelvic radiographs

Alignment
- Check the pubic symphysis is symmetrical and not widened
- Carefully check that the sacroiliac joints are intact

Bones
- Check that all three pelvic rings are intact
- Use a bright light to check iliac crests and hips
- Look at the lumbar spine and hip joints separately

Cartilage
- Check the distance of the pubic symphysis
- Again check the sacroiliac joints
- Check both hips

Soft tissues
- Check the soft tissue planes are symmetrical
- Look for obturator internus
- Carefully delineate the perivesical fat plane
- Make sure the gluteus medius and psoas fat planes are intact

Index